—THE—
Alexander Technique
MANUAL

A step-by-step guide to improve breathing, posture and well-being

RICHARD BRENNAN

Photography by Stephen Marwood

Little, Brown and Company
Boston • New York • Toronto • London

To all those who aspire to the gifts of exquisiteness and wonder that life holds.

A LITTLE, BROWN BOOK

First published in Great Britain in 1996
by Little, Brown and Company (UK)

ISBN 0-316-87497-3

First Edition
1 3 5 7 9 10 8 6 4 2

AN EDDISON • SADD EDITION
Edited, designed and produced by
Eddison Sadd Editions Limited
St Chad's House
148 King's Cross Road
London WC1X 9DH

Phototypeset in Garamond ITC Light using QuarkXPress on Apple Macintosh
Origination by HBM Print PTE Ltd, Singapore
Printed and bound at Oriental Press, UAE

Little, Brown and Company (UK)
Brettenham House
Lancaster Place
London WC2E 7EN

Contents

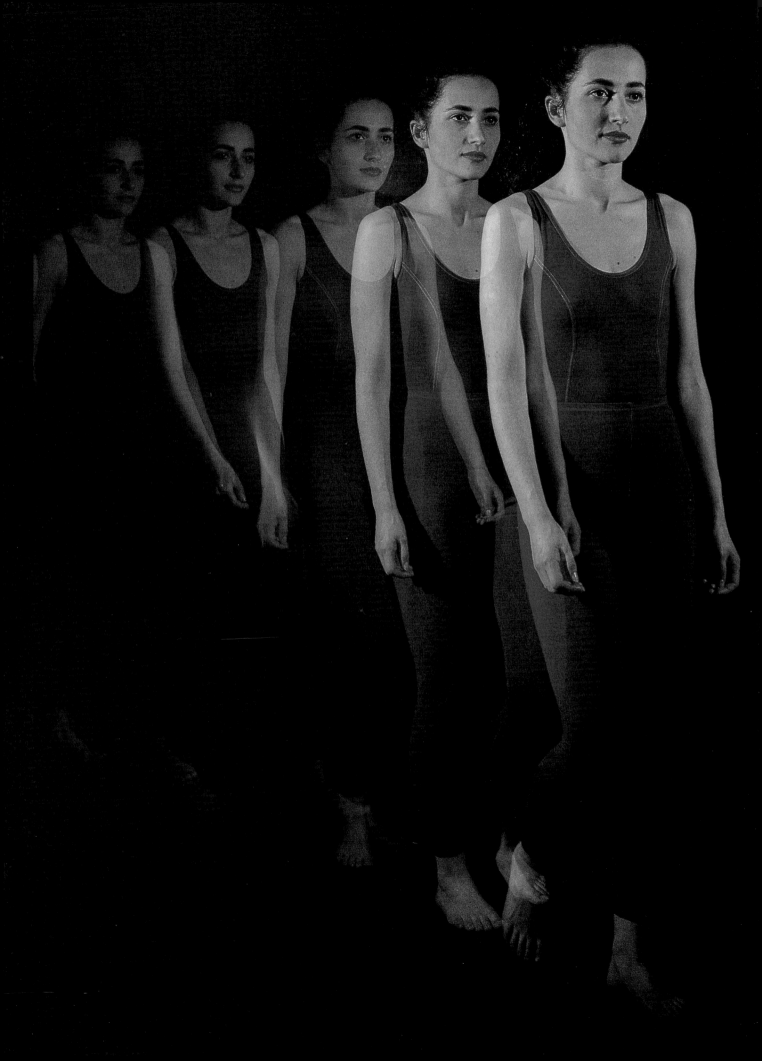

Introduction

It is often said that the trouble with the human body is that it does not come with a user's manual. Life would be much simpler if it did. This book aims to go some of the way towards fulfilling our need to understand ourselves and how we work. The Alexander Technique can help you to lead a more rewarding life, because if you use your body with more care and awareness now it will serve you well later on.

The stresses and strains of modern-day living can result in persistent muscle tension which affects our natural balance and co-ordination. This muscle tension can become chronic as a result of the mental, emotional and physical demands of life, and eventually it fixes itself within the body, distorting our physical structure and contributing to many of the health problems that are becoming increasingly prevalent in society today.

When I mention to someone that I teach the Alexander Technique, they often sit bolt upright, arching their back and pulling their shoulders back, thinking that they have now improved their posture in the way they were told to at school. They could not be further away from what the Alexander Technique is really about. Posture is far more complex than just standing or sitting up straight; it is the way in which we support and balance our bodies against the ever-present force of gravity while we go about our daily activities. In short, the human body is an amazing anti-gravity mechanism, yet most of us unconsciously interfere with its natural workings. In my opinion, this is the main reason why, for instance, millions of people throughout the Western world suffer from debilitating back pain.

Although the Alexander Technique is far reaching in its effects, it is at the same time simple in principle and can be easily understood by anyone – the only requirements are patience and a willingness to learn about yourself. By gradually becoming aware of tension and letting go of it, you will achieve a more relaxed muscular system, and this will automatically relieve or prevent many aches and pains and allow a less restricted functioning of the respiratory, circulatory and digestive systems. Since the way in which we feel physically also affects our mental and emotional outlook on life, releasing muscular tension can also help us to become more calm and generally happier in our day to day lives.

The aim of this manual is to convey the basic principles of the Technique, explain how they came about and demonstrate how you can start applying them to your own life. There is a section on pregnancy with specific advice on how the Technique can be helpful during this very important time of life, and how it can alleviate many of the aches and pains that are so often taken for granted. And the chapter on sport will help you to be aware of the way you move during various sporting activities, and also show you how you might be able to improve your performance.

The human race has explored outer space and the depths of the oceans in the quest for knowledge; now it is time for us to learn about one of the most fascinating and intriguing subjects of all – ourselves!

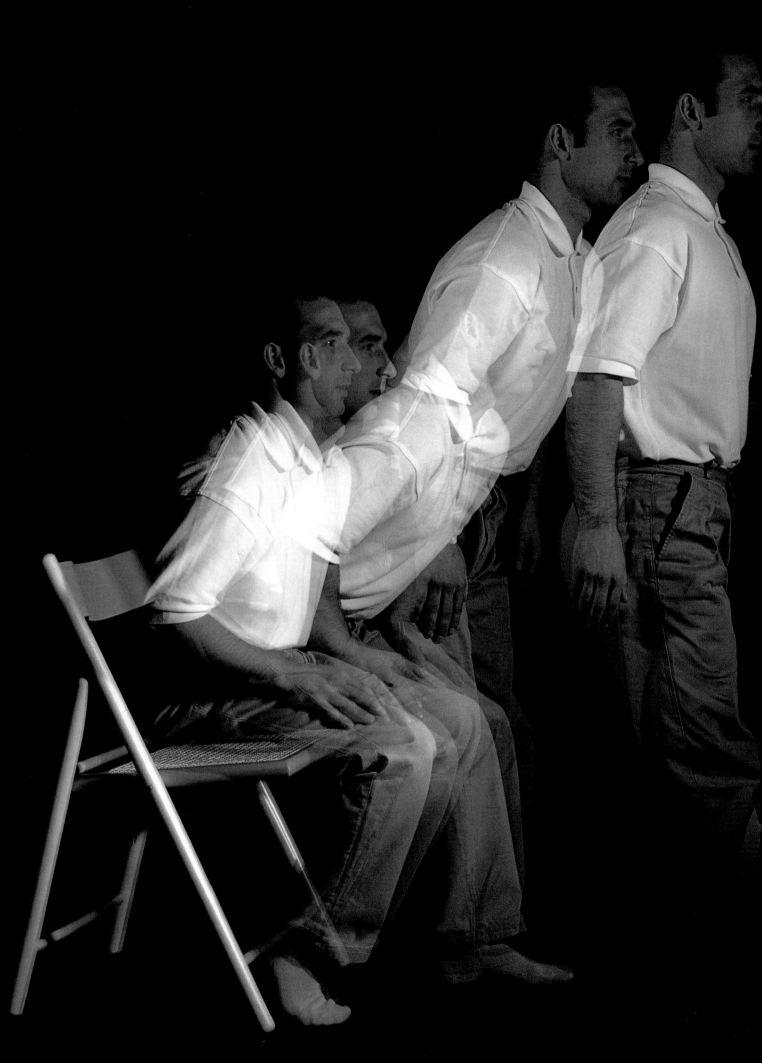

CHAPTER ONE

What is the Alexander Technique?

'*By and through consciousness and the application of a reasoning intelligence, man may rise above the powers of all disease and physical disabilities. This triumph is not to be won in sleep, in trance, in submission, in paralysis, or in anaesthesia, but in a clear, open-eyed, reasoning, deliberate consciousness and apprehension of the wonderful potentialities possessed by mankind, the transcendent inheritance of a conscious mind.*'

Frederick Matthias Alexander

Even a simple action such as getting up from a chair can be detrimental to the neck and spine as many of us unconsciously throw our head back on to our spine with great force. By allowing the head to go forwards and upwards, this man is able to get up with the minimum amount of effort, which not only prevents harmful muscular tension but also encourages easy and graceful movement.

What is the Alexander Technique?

The Alexander Technique is not so much something you learn as something you unlearn. It is a method of releasing unwanted muscular tension throughout your body which has accumulated over many years of stressful living. This excess tension often starts in childhood and, if left unchecked, can give rise in later life to common ailments such as arthritis, neck and back pain, migraines, hypertension, sciatica, insomnia and even depression. Vast amounts of money are being spent on the treatment of these illnesses (to say nothing of the pain and discomfort that is endured by the sufferer), yet the number of patients continues to increase. With the right education, however, many people could be helped to understand the causes of their problems and be taught to help themselves, so that their aches and pains may either be relieved or avoided altogether.

The Alexander Technique can help us to become more aware of balance, posture and co-ordination while performing everyday actions. This brings into consciousness tensions throughout our body that have previously gone unnoticed, and it is these tensions which are very often the root cause of many common ailments. This is exactly what Frederick Matthias Alexander, the originator of the Technique, discovered when trying to get to the bottom of his own voice-related problem. You can read about how he came to his conclusions later on in this chapter (see page 18).

When applying the Alexander Technique you will learn how to release unnecessary muscle tension. As most of this tension has built up very gradually over a number of years you are unlikely to be aware that it is even there at all. You will also learn new ways of moving while carrying out everyday actions which cause far less strain on the body, and discover ways of sitting, standing and walking that put less strain on the bones, joints and muscles, thus making your body work more efficiently. In fact, many people who practise the Technique experience a general feeling of lightness throughout their bodies and even describe the sensation as being like 'walking on air'. Since our physical state directly affects both our mental and emotional well-being, people often say that they feel much calmer and happier even after just a few Alexander lessons. This often results in less domestic tension and a greater ability to cope with life in general.

The Alexander Technique also involves examining posture, breathing, balance and co-ordination. As children, our posture and ease of movement are a joy to watch, but as we start to tense our muscles in reaction to many of life's worries and concerns, our posture deteriorates into what can border on deformity. Yet this is not the case with people outside Western civilization – many of the indigenous races who still live on the land, such as Native Americans, the Berber people from North Africa and the Aborigines in Australia, retain their natural posture throughout their lives (see opposite). Their upright posture is considered to be a reflection of their human dignity and integrity.

We have a series of reflexes throughout the body that support us and naturally co-ordinate our movements, yet we interfere with these natural reflexes to such an extent that many of us often hold four or five times more tension in our bodies than is really necessary. In fact, we often make life much harder for ourselves than it really needs to be, although of course we are completely unaware that this is the case. Our shoulders become permanently hunched, our necks become stiffer and stiffer, and we sit either slumped or holding ourselves in a very rigid fashion, as our minds become more and more concerned with the future and the past and our awareness of the 'present moment' diminishes.

Over the years we become accustomed to the ways in which we sit and stand, without realizing that it is often these very positions

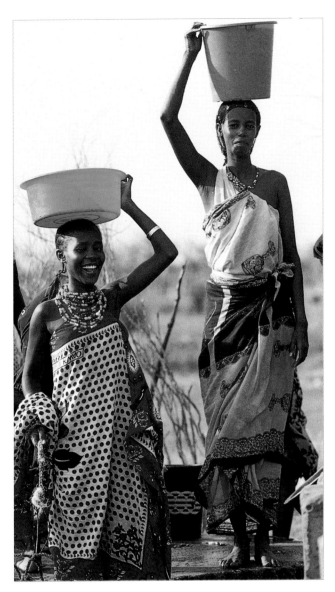

Poor posture is not a necessary part of being an adult. These African women maintain their poise and ease of movement (inherent in every small child) throughout their lives. This, in turn, has a positive bearing on their sense of well-being.

painkilling drugs that block out the body's warning system, whose function it is to tell us that something is wrong. Often, doctors can offer little advice as their training revolves around the treating of symptoms rather than uncovering, and also rectifying, the causes of such problems. The Alexander Technique, however, does just this; it shows you the underlying cause, so enabling you to eliminate the tension responsible for so many of the ailments that we mistakenly put down to the ageing process.

This is illustrated by the true story of a sixty-five-year-old lady whose left leg gave her a great deal of pain whenever she stood or walked on it. She approached her doctor who sent her for tests and an X-ray. When the results came through the doctor told her that she had arthritis and it was simply caused by old age. She refused to believe that the reason was simply age alone, since, as she pointed out to her doctor, her right leg was perfectly alright and both her legs were the same age! She was obviously putting excessive strain on the leg that was causing problems, and if she could work out how she was doing this she would be able to go some way towards alleviating the pain in her leg.

Back pain

One of the most common examples of stress-related illness is back pain. Eighty per cent of all people living in the West will suffer from disabling lower back pain at some point in their lives. In the United States 100 million visits are made to chiropractors each year, and in the UK 60 million working days are lost each year because of back trouble, and these figures are doubling every decade. Up to eighty per cent of Americans will have had some type of lower back problem by the age of fifty, and it has been estimated that over 230,000 people in the UK alone are off work with backache every day. This figure does not account for all those who do not work – nor does it include many more people who have backache, but still carry on working. The actual number of people who suffer with back

that are putting strains upon our body – no matter how uncoordinated these positions are, they will always feel right to us. When we perform everyday activities it is amazing how frequently we subject our bodies to undue tension simply by not being aware of what we are doing; this tension spreads throughout the muscular system, even if it is triggered in one particular area of the body *(see overleaf)*.

It may be many years before we start to suffer from aches and pains or restriction of movement. Many of our modern methods of combating such problems involve powerful

11

pain could well exceed 20 million, which is staggering when you realize that this is equal to nearly a third of the UK population.

Throughout the Western world the statistics reveal that back pain is not confined only to the United States and England, but seems to be on the increase in most developed countries, yet few people seem to have any clear answers or solutions to the problem. Although a great deal of money is being spent on treating back pain, and the treatments themselves often have unpleasant side effects, there is little research into why it is so prevalent in our society but comparatively rare in some underdeveloped countries. Doctors, back specialists and orthopaedic surgeons openly admit that the cause of back pain is often a mystery and after surgery many people suffer with even greater discomfort than before. The same can be said for other common ailments, such as arthritis or headaches.

Taking responsibility

Many people carry on for years enduring unnecessary pain, not realizing that anything can be done for them. We need to face up to the fact that we have to take responsibility for our ailments and not expect other people to have all the answers. After all, the reasons for many of these problems can be found when we consider our own posture and the way we use our body while performing even the simplest of tasks: pain is simply the body's warning system trying to tell us that something is going wrong. If you were driving a car and the oil light came on, you would not take out the bulb and carry on driving; this, of course, would be foolish. You would stop the car, try to find out what was wrong and attempt to fix it; otherwise it might result in more serious problems later on. This is exactly what we should be doing with our own bodies, yet most

Below. *Notice how uncoordinated this woman's movements are during the simple action of turning on a light – her legs are going in one direction, yet the rest of her body is going in another. This is causing her to distort her whole body, which in turn results in excessive muscular tension throughout her body.*

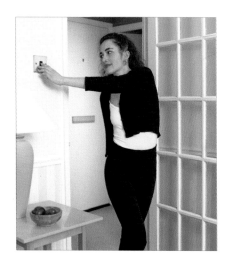

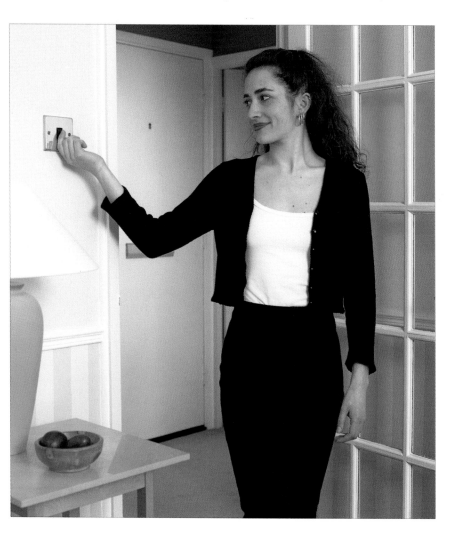

Right. *Simply by using the hand which is nearer the light switch she is able to perform the same action with more efficiency and a great deal less stress on her body as a whole – it also looks more graceful.*

Below. *The way this woman is loading the washing machine is putting her muscles under an enormous strain. Notice how most of her body weight is in front of her feet causing her neck, back and leg muscles to be excessively tense in order to prevent her from falling forward.*

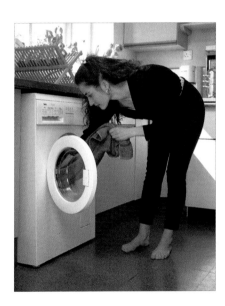

Right. *Simply by squatting down to do the same activity it allows her entire body to be in balance because most of her body weight is now above her feet. If she regularly adopts this posture when bending down she will be less likely to suffer from back pain.*

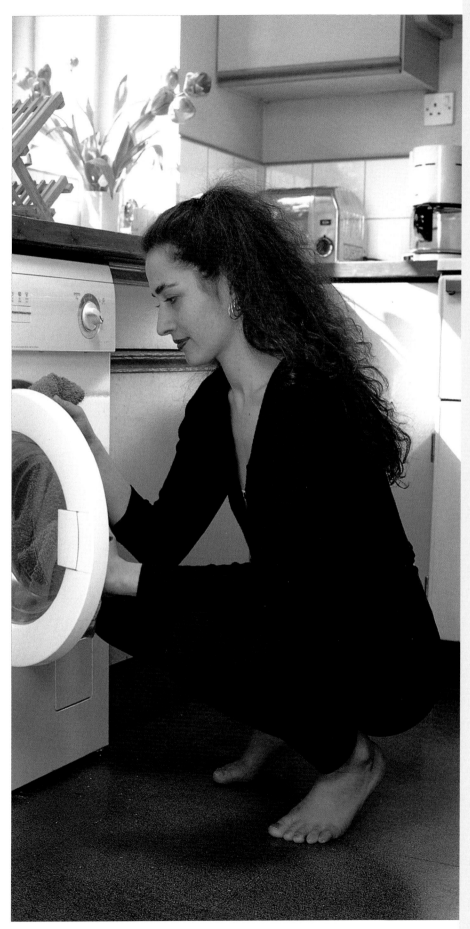

13

of us try to eliminate pain without investigating what is causing it in the first place.

When applying the Alexander Technique as a daily practice you will be able to make conscious choices which surpass the physical realm and this will allow you to have more freedom in every aspect of your life. Since the physical postures we tend to adopt are merely a reflection of our inner selves (for example, if you are depressed or fed up you are likely to hang your head down slightly and adopt a slumped posture), many people find that they are also breaking mental and emotional habits that have been present for most of their life. It is important to realize that only the behaviour patterns no longer serving you will be eliminated, and this enables you to express yourself without fear of judgement or criticism. The Technique is a tool by which you can gain a real freedom of choice and this will naturally lead to a more harmonious and happier way of life. Indeed, it is for this very reason that the Alexander Technique is often thought of as a philosophy for living.

Alexander lessons

Although the Alexander Technique is, in essence, simple, it is often extremely difficult to see your own habits and places of tension within your body, so finding a teacher is particularly important to help you through the difficulties that can arise during the learning process. In this book you will learn about the principles and the philosophy behind the Alexander Technique, but it is not a substitute for actual lessons from a qualified teacher: after all, you would not expect to drive a car after only having read a teach-yourself-to-drive book. However, once you have grasped the principles of the Technique discussed in this book, you will be able to understand more quickly and easily what your teacher is trying to convey, which can save you both time and money.

Many people ask me whether they are too old to learn the Technique. In my opinion, the answer is no – I have taught people well into their eighties who have made remarkable

THE THREE STAGES OF LEARNING THE TECHNIQUE

1. Releasing unwanted tension that has accumulated over many years of standing or sitting in an uncoordinated manner.
2. Learning new ways of moving, standing or sitting that are easier, more efficient and put less stress on the body. This reduces excessive wear and tear on the bones and joints and also allows all the internal organs sufficient space to function naturally.
3. Learning new ways of reacting physically, emotionally and mentally to various situations.

progress. It must be said, though, that the younger you are, the fewer habits you will have accumulated and so it is likely that you will be able to release tensions more quickly. Having said this, the main requirements, no matter what age you are, are patience and a willingness to learn about yourself and the ingrained habits that you have acquired throughout your life.

Alexander Technique lessons last for anywhere between half an hour and an hour. During this time your teacher will move your limbs, head and body through various postures so that he or she can detect any areas where you may be holding muscular tension *(see opposite)*. The process is very gentle and painless. When tension is discovered, your teacher will ask you to let go of it, and you will be amazed at the difference that you will feel after only a few lessons.

Although the Alexander Technique is often grouped with other complementary health subjects such as osteopathy or homeopathy, it is really quite different in that it teaches people ways of helping themselves, so that in the future they begin to know naturally what to do if any aches or pains arise. Although Alexander lessons do have therapeutic results, the practitioner is called a teacher rather than a therapist, as the student is given full responsibility for their own well-being; it is up to them to practise what they have learned between lessons. Alexander Technique lessons are discussed in more detail in chapter eight.

14

Awareness

The key to learning the Technique is awareness. At first, being aware of how we perform various tasks seems very alien, because we are used to moving automatically without any thought whatsoever. Slowly, we are taught to think for a moment before performing any given action to see how it can be carried out with the minimum of tension *(see overleaf)*.

Most people are surprised when they find out that they are causing their neck or back muscles to tense needlessly. By analysing even simple movements, such as walking or getting up from a chair, we can find new ways of moving that release tension rather

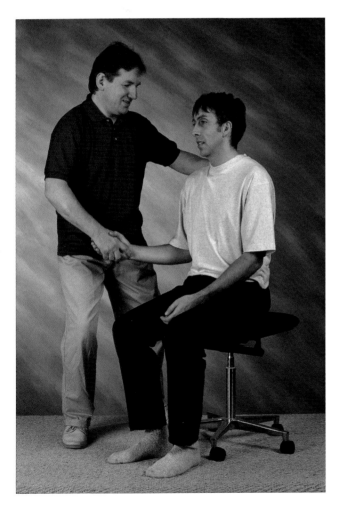

During your Alexander Technique lessons, your teacher will gently move your head and limbs in order to detect any muscular tension within your body. When the teacher feels some resistance, he or she will make you aware of the tension so that you can let it go. With practice, you will find that you can release this tension on your own.

than create it. People who have undergone a course of lessons generally feel less tired and have more energy to do the things they enjoy, instead of sitting around each evening feeling too exhausted to do anything. In this way the quality of their lives is greatly enhanced and feelings of calmness, happiness and a greater sense of well-being often come to the fore.

We rarely pay much attention to ourselves apart from when it comes to our appearance – we may well spend a lot of money on clothes, make-up and perfume trying to make ourselves more attractive and yet there is nothing more beautiful than someone who is moving gracefully or standing with poise. Many people who have taken lessons say that the Technique has helped them to look and feel years younger, which is something nearly everyone would like to achieve! In addition, it will help you not only to be more aware of your body, but also of the world about you. You will find that you have a greater appreciation of life in general, as many worries and concerns begin to fade.

Re-education

When you begin to apply the principles of the Technique you will not be learning to do anything new, but simply unlearning many habits that you have acquired during the course of your life. Alexander himself often said that if you stopped doing the wrong thing (the habit) then the right thing would happen by itself. It is, however, sometimes harder to relearn something than it is to learn it in the first place, because our normal way of performing actions feels so right. But as you start to allow tension to release you will find that you are naturally using your body in a much more balanced and co-ordinated way. Any aches or pains should slowly begin to ease, and eventually disappear altogether.

It is important to realize that the whole process of re-evaluating the way in which you move does take time, as you are dealing with habits that have been present since childhood. As the pace of life increases it seems that we often expect results immediately, and

15

Below. *Simple everyday activities such as speaking on the phone can cause unnecessary stress. Notice how this woman is using her shoulder to hold the phone; this posture, if repeated often enough, becomes habitual and can lead to chronic shoulder or neck pain.*

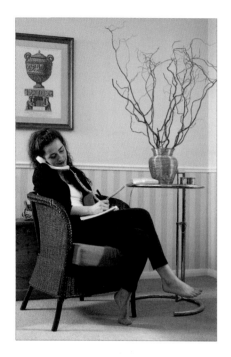

Right. *When a little thought is given to the way we perform common tasks, such as holding a phone or writing, we are able to adopt new ways of moving that help to keep the body in alignment. Simple changes, such as holding the phone in your hand and writing on a table instead of on your knee, help your posture to improve naturally. This helps to prevent your muscles from being in a permanently tense state and can also improve your breathing.*

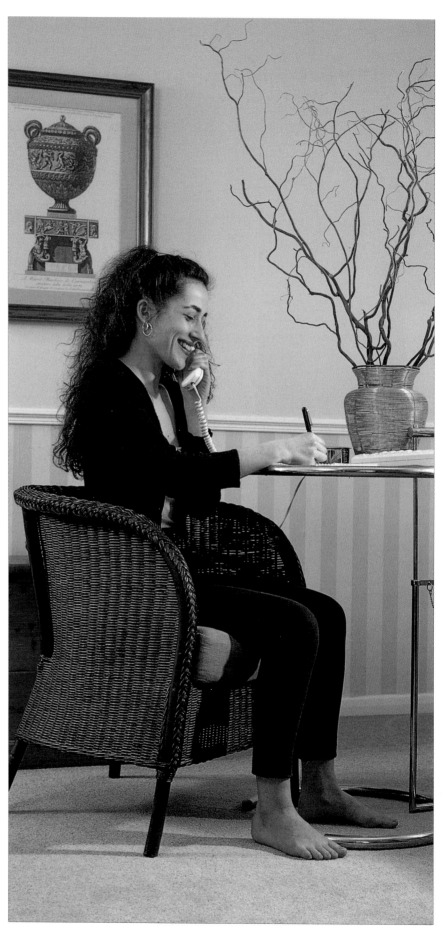

yet nature is not like that. It will take time for the body to restructure itself and it may even take a few lessons just to comprehend what is being asked of you.

Changing your patterns of behaviour

Throughout our lives we all develop physical, mental and emotional patterns of behaviour; usually other people are more aware of them than we are ourselves. We react to a given situation over and over again in the same way, regardless of whether or not it is appropriate, and as many of these reactions are unconscious, we will repeat them time after time without being aware of it. In fact, most of these ways of responding were learnt as a child and some began even before our earliest childhood memory.

A good example of habitual behaviour can be seen when we are running late for an appointment. Many of us react physically by hunching our shoulders; we no longer think rationally and, if driving a car, we may take unnecessary risks as we fear the consequences of being late, even when the appointment is of little importance, such as meeting a friend for a drink. We may even risk our lives trying to get to work on time! These emotional, physical and mental reactions often become ingrained during our school days, when being late might result in some form of ridicule or punishment.

How the Technique can help you

There are a number of different reasons for taking up Alexander Technique lessons, and the most motivating one is pain. I myself used to suffer from acute sciatica; I sought help from doctors, chiropractors, an osteopath and numerous physiotherapists but nothing at all seemed to help. In fact, some of the treatment even seemed to make my condition worse! I started to have Alexander lessons, and discovered that my sciatica was partly caused by sitting in an awkward position for long periods while I was teaching people to drive. When I changed the way I sat and moved, the

muscle that was trapping the sciatic nerve released, and the shooting pain down my legs also ceased.

Here are some common examples of when the Alexander Technique could help you in your day to day life:

• You may be one of those millions of people who regularly suffer from backache, a stiff neck, headaches, arthritis or other symptoms for which there seems to be no answer. The Alexander Technique does not set out to cure the specific symptoms of these ailments, but it does help you to uncover and change the harmful and unconscious habitual patterns which can all too often be the underlying cause of your problem.

• You may be suffering from stress as a result of work, or perhaps for domestic reasons. The Technique will help you look more closely at your reactions in everyday situations, and enable you to see for yourself how you contribute to the build-up of excessive tension in your life. By changing the way you react to various situations you can drastically reduce your stress levels, so possibly avoiding high blood pressure, stomach ulcers or even heart attacks and strokes.

• You may be suffering from pain or discomfort without knowing why. The Technique can help you to see that it could well be your postural habits that are the root cause of your problem.

• You may be pregnant and want to look after your body in order to give both your baby and yourself the best chance of a healthy pregnancy and an easier and more natural birth (see chapter seven).

• You may be a musician, actor, dancer, singer or sportsperson (for sports see chapter six), who relies on their body to function at its peak efficiency. The Alexander Technique will provide you with a means of releasing excessive tension, enabling you to perform much closer to your maximum ability with minimum effort. It is interesting to note that many of the main music and drama colleges now include the Alexander Technique as part of their curriculum.

• You may already be perfectly healthy, but simply want to take more responsibility for your own health and sense of well-being, as indeed do an ever-increasing number of people today. You might want to discover more about yourself, or wish to use the Alexander Technique to prevent ill health in later life. I teach many people in their forties and fifties, for instance, who tell me that they wish they had known about the Technique twenty years ago.

These are only some of the more common applications, and in fact the Technique can be used by practically anyone to improve the functioning of their entire body. The benefits are enormous – not only physically, but mentally and emotionally as well. You have so much to gain and so little to lose.

THE ALEXANDER TECHNIQUE IS …

• *A way of becoming aware and letting go of tension throughout your body.*
• *A re-education, so that you learn how to use your body in a more appropriate way, and avoid putting stress on the bones, joints and internal organs.*
• *A process by which you get to know yourself better, not only physically but also mentally and emotionally as well.*
• *A way of making real choices in your life, rather than reacting habitually to any given situation.*
• *A way of understanding how the body is naturally designed to work, and learning how to stop interfering with these natural functions.*
• *A technique which you can practise, with the help of lessons, that can bring about harmony and contentment in your life.*

In order to understand the Alexander Technique fully, it is important to comprehend the various stages that Alexander himself had to go through in order to develop it. The entire process took place over a seven-year period, and he constantly revised the Technique right up to the time of his death over sixty years after the initial discovery. Even today the Technique is continually being developed by trained Alexander teachers who are discovering how important Alexander's initial findings were.

Evolution of a technique

Frederick Matthias Alexander was born in Australia on 20 January 1869, the eldest of the eight children of John and Betsy Alexander. He grew up in a small town called Wynyard, situated on the north-west coast of the island of Tasmania. Frederick was born prematurely, and without his mother's overwhelming love for her child he would not have survived more than a few weeks (she was, in fact, the local nurse and midwife).

Frederick was a very sickly child, suffering from asthma and other respiratory problems. Due to his frail health, he was taken away from school at an early age and was tutored in the evenings by the local school teacher. During the day he helped his father look after the horses, and this could have accounted for the sensitivity in his hands, which was later to play a crucial part in the teaching of his Technique to others.

During his teenage years Frederick's health gradually improved, and by the time he was seventeen financial pressures within the family had forced him to leave the outdoor life of which he had become so fond to work in the Mount Bischoff Tin Mining Company. When not at work he taught himself to play the violin, and also took part in amateur dramatics. At the age of twenty he had saved up enough money to enable him to travel to Melbourne, where he stayed with his uncle, James Pearce, and passed the next three months spending his hard-earned savings on going to the theatre and concerts and visiting art galleries. At the end of this three-month period Alexander had firmly decided to train to be an actor and reciter.

Voice problems

Alexander stayed on in Melbourne and took on a variety of jobs, working for an estate agent, in a department store and even as a tea-taster for a tea merchant to finance his training, which he did in the evenings and at weekends. It was not long before he gained a fine reputation at a first-class reciter, and went on to form his own theatre company which specialized in one-man Shakespeare recitals.

As he became increasingly successful, Alexander began to accept more and more engagements, which in turn put greater strain on his vocal cords. Within a short time the stress began to show, as his voice regularly became hoarse in the middle of his performances. He approached several doctors and voice trainers who gave him medication and suggested exercises, but nothing seemed to make any difference. In fact, the situation deteriorated further still, until on one occasion Alexander could barely finish his recital. He became increasingly anxious as he realized that his entire career was in jeopardy. He approached yet another doctor, who was convinced that the vocal cords had merely been over-strained and prescribed complete rest of his voice for two weeks, promising that this would give Alexander a solution to his problem. Determined to try anything, Alexander uttered hardly a word for the two-week period preceding his next important engagement.

At the beginning of the performance he was delighted to find that his voice was crystal clear; in fact, it was better than it had been for months. This soon turned to dismay, however, when half-way through his performance the hoarseness in his voice returned, and his condition continued to deteriorate until by the end of the evening he could hardly speak. The next day, feeling very disappointed, he returned to his doctor and reported what had happened. The doctor felt that his treatment had had some effect and advised a longer period of rest for the vocal cords. What transpired next proved to be at the very heart of the Alexander Technique.

Cause and effect

Alexander refused any further treatment, stating that after two weeks of following the doctor's instructions implicitly his problem had returned within the hour. Alexander then reasoned with the doctor that if his voice was perfect when he started the recital, and yet was in a terrible state by the time he had finished, it must have been something that he

was doing while performing that was in fact causing the problem. The doctor thought carefully for a moment and then agreed that this must be the case. 'Can you tell me, then, what it was that caused the trouble?' Alexander asked. The doctor admitted honestly that he did not know.

Alexander left the surgery determined to find a solution to his curious problem. This took him on a journey of discovery that not only gave him the answer to his question, but also revealed the mechanics of movement of the human being and the interference with these reflexes that contributes to much of our suffering in modern civilization. Alexander's findings were greatly underestimated at the time, although his discovery has now come to be regarded as one of the greatest of the twentieth century.

You may be thinking that you do not have a problem with your voice, but it is your back, neck, shoulders or another part of your body that hurts. The point is that Alexander's logic can be applied to practically any ailment we have. For example, if your back is fine before you do the gardening, yet you have back pain afterwards, then it must follow that you are putting your body under undue stress while digging or weeding and this is the underlying cause of your problem. It does not matter what physical ailment you are suffering from; there is always a reason behind the problem, and when that reason is removed the pain or discomfort will gradually disappear.

Initial investigations

Alexander had only two clues to follow up when he started his investigations:

1. The act of reciting on stage brought about the hoarseness which caused him to lose his voice.
2. When speaking in a normal manner, the hoarseness in his voice disappeared.

Following simple, logical steps Alexander deduced that if ordinary speaking did not cause him to lose his voice, whereas reciting did, there must be something different about what he did when doing one or the other. If he could find out what that difference was, he might be able to change the way in which he was using his voice when reciting, which would then solve his problem. He used a mirror to observe himself both when speaking in his normal voice and again when reciting, in the hope that he could discern certain differences between the two. He watched carefully, but could see nothing wrong or unnatural while speaking normally. It was when he began to recite that he noticed several actions that were different:

• He tended to pull his head back on to his spine with a certain amount of force.
• He simultaneously depressed his larynx (the cavity in the throat where the vocal cords are situated).
• He correspondingly began to suck in air through his mouth, so producing a gasping sound.

Up until this point Alexander had been completely unaware of these habits, and when he returned to his normal speaking voice he realized that the same tendencies were still present but to a lesser extent. This was the reason why they had previously gone undetected. So, Alexander's first discovery was: **misuse of the body often occurs habitually and unconsciously.**

He returned to the mirror with new encouragement and recited over and over again to see if he could find any more clues. He soon noticed that the three tendencies became accentuated when he was reading passages in which unusual demands were made on his voice. This confirmed his earlier suspicion that there was definitely some sort of connection between the way in which he recited and his loss of voice. It dawned on him for the first time that he was unconsciously causing his own problem.

The primary control
The next stumbling block Alexander encountered was that he was unsure of what was responsible for causing these damaging tendencies. He found himself in a maze of questions: was it the sucking in of air while breathing that caused him to pull back his head and depress his larynx? Or was it the pulling back of his head that caused him to depress his larynx and suck in air? Or was it the depression of his larynx that caused him to suck in air and pull back his head?

At first he was unable to answer these questions, but he went on experimenting patiently in front of the mirror. After some months he realized that he could not directly prevent the sucking in of air while breathing or the depression of the larynx, but he could to some extent prevent the pulling back of his head by releasing muscle tension. When he did this he also noticed that it indirectly improved the state of his larynx and his breathing. At this point Alexander wrote in his journal:

'The importance of this discovery cannot be over-estimated, for through it I was led on to the further discovery of the primary control of the working of all the mechanisms of the human organism, and this marked the first important stage of my investigation.'

Alexander had made his second discovery: **the existence of the primary control (the dynamic relationship of the head to the spine), which allows for optimal activity of the muscles and reflexes throughout the rest of the body.**

Alexander carried on with his experiments, and soon found that when he prevented himself from pulling his head back the hoarseness in his voice decreased. He returned to his doctor, who found that there had been a considerable improvement in the general condition of his throat and vocal cords. Alexander now had positive proof that the manner in which he was reciting was causing him to lose his voice, and that changing the way in which he performed would eventually lead to an eradication of his problem. Alexander's third discovery was therefore: **the way in which the body is used will invariably affect all of its various functions.**

Faulty sensory perception

Enthused with the idea that he was at last getting to the crux of the matter, Alexander experimented further still to see if he could achieve even greater improvement in the state of his vocal cords. He did this by deliberately putting his head forward, but was surprised to find that this also had the effect of depressing his larynx. In order to have a closer look at how he was moving, he added two further mirrors on either side of the original one. When he observed himself again in the mirrors, he could see clearly that he was in fact still pulling his head down on to his spine as before. Alexander was very surprised at these findings, because he realized that he was doing the exact *opposite* of what he thought he was doing. He had just made his next discovery: **he was suffering from a faulty sensory awareness.**

In other words, he could no longer rely on his sensory feeling to tell him what he was or was not doing. At first he thought that this was his own personal idiosyncrasy, but when he started to teach his Technique he found that faulty sensory perception was practically universal. Feeling disillusioned, yet unable to give up his quest, Alexander persevered and began to notice that his habit of pulling his head back and down was not only causing the depression of his larynx, but also causing various tensions and stresses throughout his entire body. He became aware that he was also lifting his chest, arching his back, throwing his pelvis forward, over-tightening his leg muscles and even gripping the floor with his feet. This was affecting his balance and also the way in which he moved. This led him to his next discovery: **the body does not function as separate entities, but as a whole unit with every part affecting every other part.**

During his training he had been taught to 'take hold of the floor' with his feet by one of his recital tutors. He had obeyed by tensing his feet and toes, believing that his teacher obviously knew better than him. Similarly, in our society we are told to sit or stand in a certain way in order to correct poor posture. Even if we achieve what we imagine people are asking of us, we can actually be making the situation worse instead of better. This is because we are under the illusion that other people know what good posture is, when in fact they do not.

It then dawned on Alexander that the tightening of all the muscles in his legs and feet was part of the same habit that was causing him to tighten his neck muscles. The action of 'taking hold of the floor' with his feet had, over the years, become such an ingrained habit that he was completely unaware that he was doing it. He found it almost impossible to recite without all his habits being present, and whatever he did to change the way he recited simply increased the amount of tension, and this ultimately made things worse. So, Alexander's next discovery was: **a given stimulus produces the same reaction over and over again which, if it goes unchecked, turns into habitual behaviour. This habitual reaction feels normal and natural to us.**

Alexander now found himself in an impossible situation, because he was relying on his sensory feelings to give him information, yet he already knew from previous experience that he could not rely on these feelings. At this stage in his experiments he wrote in his journal:

> *'It is important to remember that the use of a specific part in any activity is closely associated with the use of other parts of the organism, and that the influence exerted by the various parts one upon another is continuously changing in accordance with the manner of the use of these parts. If a part directly employed in the activity is being used in a comparatively new way which is still unfamiliar, the stimulus to use this part in the new way is weak in comparison with the stimulus to use the other parts of the organism, which are being indirectly employed in the activity, in the old habitual way.'*

Alexander went on to say that, in his case, an attempt was being made to bring about an

21

unfamiliar use of his head and neck for the purpose of reciting. The stimulus to employ the new use of his head and neck was therefore bound to be weak, as compared with the stimulus to employ the habitual (yet wrong) use of his feet and legs which had become familiar through being cultivated in the act of reciting. This is where the difficulty lies – in breaking our old habits to learn new ways of functioning.

Directions

This led Alexander on to the whole question of how he consciously directed himself while reciting. He realized that he never gave any thought to how he moved, but simply moved in a way that was habitual because it felt 'right' to him. At first he tried to correct himself by actually putting his head forward and upward, but soon found that this once again increased the very muscular tension that he was trying to eliminate. At this point he gave up in exasperation and almost at once achieved the release of tension he had wanted. He realized that he merely had to *think* of the directions in order to bring about a change without creating further tension, and he began to experiment with being aware of what he was doing and consciously directing the way in which he moved. He described this process as *thinking in activity*.

The meaning of the word 'directing', as Alexander used it, is consciously to give a mental order to your body, so that your body will respond to what you tell it to do rather than working by habit alone. For example, when a person realizes that their shoulders are hunched they think of releasing the tension and their shoulders immediately drop. A more detailed explanation of this can be found in chapter four.

When Alexander had practised his directions for long enough he decided to return to the mirrors and try out his new findings during the action of reciting. To his dismay, he found that he failed far more often than he succeeded. He was sure that he had found the answer to his problem, but began to believe that it was his own personal shortcoming that

prevented him from achieving his objectives. He looked around for all possible causes of failure and after many months saw that he was giving his directions successfully right up to the time of speaking but was then immediately reverting back to his old habitual way of pulling his head back and causing tension throughout his body. Alexander had been so goal-orientated when it came to reciting that any attempts to 'get it right' had resulted in tension in his neck muscles. He had to find a way of not caring whether he achieved his end. He worked out the following plan:

ALEXANDER'S PLAN

1. He would inhibit any immediate response to the stimulus to speak the sentence.
2. He would use his new directions, which would allow him to achieve less tension in his neck and throat.
3. He would continue to project these directions until he was familiar enough with them to apply them consistently whilst reciting.
4. While still continuing to give his directions he would ask himself whether he should:
a) go ahead and perform his task of reciting
b) choose not to speak after all
c) choose to do something different altogether.

After working on this plan for some time, Alexander devised his Technique, which primarily consists of awareness, eradication of harmful habits and free choice. He was able not only to free himself from the habit which had jeopardized his career, but also to cure himself of the recurring asthma that had afflicted him from birth.

Interest grows

When Alexander returned to the stage, many of his fellow actors who were suffering from similar problems sought his help, and he began teaching his Technique to others. News spread like wildfire about the actor who had cured himself of his vocal and respiratory difficulties and doctors began referring some of their patients to Alexander, who had enormous success in treating a variety of ailments.

He used the gentle guidance of his hands, as well as verbal instructions, to convey his Technique. He helped many people release the harmful habits which were at the root of their illnesses.

One of the doctors, Dr J. W. Stewart McKay, could see the great potential in his work and persuaded Alexander to go to London in order to bring the Technique to a wider audience. In the spring of 1904 Alexander set sail for England. He arrived later that year and set up a practice in Victoria Street, and later at Ashley Place in central London. Alexander was soon regarded by many as a 'cult' figure; he taught a number of famous people of that period, including George Bernard Shaw, Aldous Huxley, Sir Henry Irving (actor), John Dewey (philosopher and educationalist) and Sir Charles Sherrington (Nobel prizewinner for physiology and medicine). In his early sixties, he was encouraged to set up a teacher training course for fear that his Technique would die with him, and in 1931 he started to train teachers at his home in Ashley Place. He continued teaching privately, as well as training new teachers, right up until his death in the October of 1955.

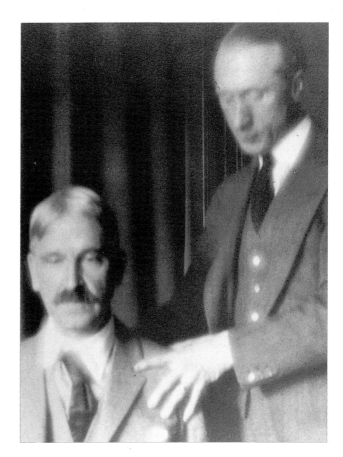

This is Frederick Matthias Alexander giving one of his pupils a lesson – here he is encouraging a widening of the man's shoulder. Notice his gentle and unimposing touch, which in turn affects his pupil's entire muscular system.

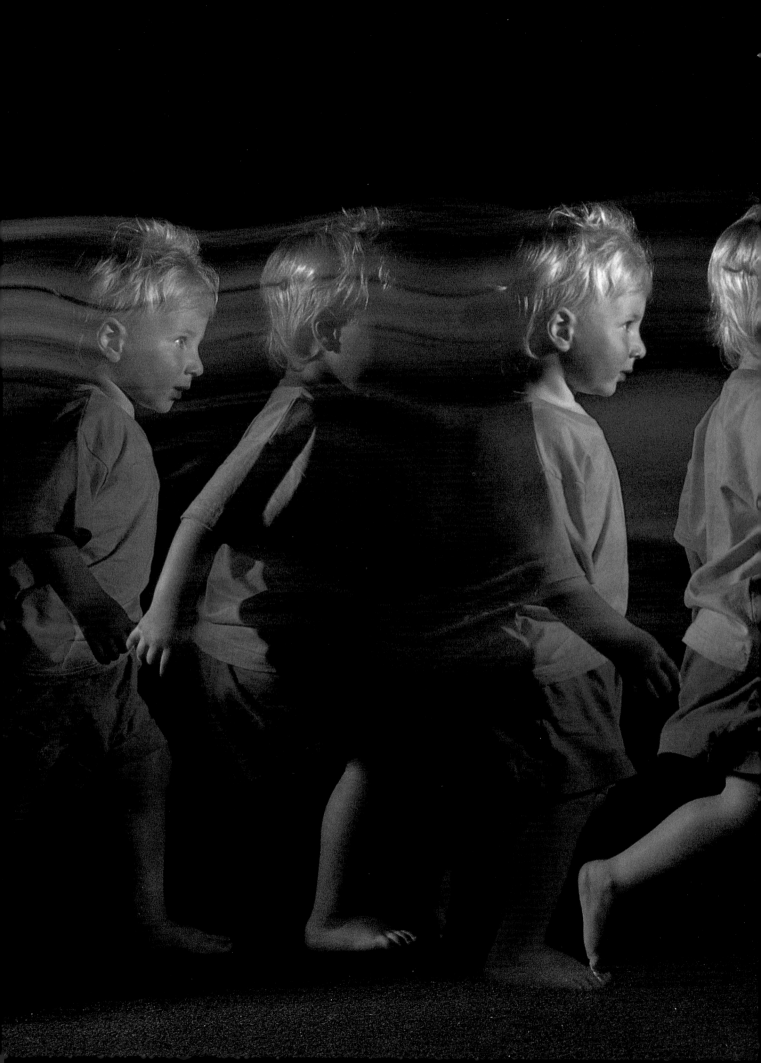

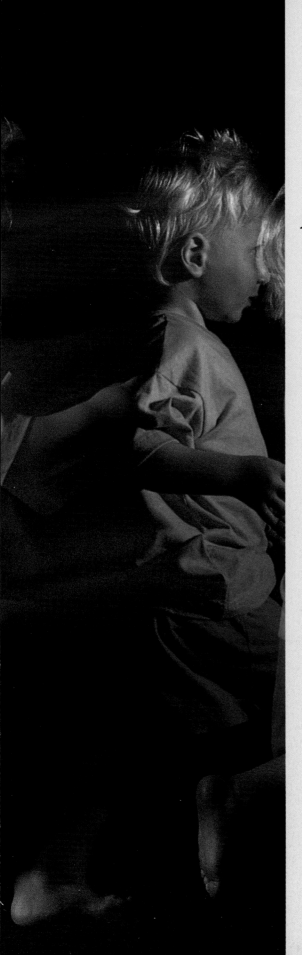

CHAPTER TWO

How the Alexander Technique is relevant to you

'By emerging from the contest with nature he [man] has ceased to be a natural animal. He has evolved curious powers of discrimination, of choice, and of construction. He has changed his environment, his food, and his whole manner of living. He has inquired into laws which govern heredity and into the causes of disease. But still his knowledge is limited, and his emergence incomplete. The power of the force we know as evolution still holds him in chains, though man has loosened his bonds and may at last free himself entirely.'

Frederick Matthias Alexander

Children move with minimum effort – notice how this boy's head leads his movements and the rest of his body follows naturally with ease. As adults, our movements are often uncoordinated; the Alexander Technique helps us to learn new ways of moving and rediscover our natural grace and poise for a healthier and happier lifestyle.

How the Alexander Technique is relevant to you

Although we have made great medical and scientific advances over the last century and have conquered many serious diseases, there are many other forms of illness and doctors and scientists can do little to stop these reaching epidemic proportions. These include backache, neck and shoulder pains, arthritis, spinal diseases (spondylitis, scoliosis, multiple sclerosis), asthma, depression, various neuroses (such as panic attacks or phobias) and insomnia. Very few of these are fatal, but they adversely affect the quality of life of the sufferer and his or her family. Such conditions invariably lead to unhappiness and stress, and also restrict the person's ability to perform various activities.

Although the answers to many of these problems are researched in laboratories, the solution is not to be found there. Initially, great hope for the sufferer is promised by the numerous drugs that come on to the market each year, but unfortunately hopes are often dashed as the body becomes immune to the drug's effect. Instead, the explanation for the huge majority of common complaints is to be found in the way we live our lives, and this is where the Alexander Technique can play such an important part – it is up to us to take positive action to help ourselves.

Life is not an emergency

Life seems to be forever moving at an increasingly faster pace. Many people who are in full-time employment are continually under pressure as they try to meet impossible deadlines. The result of this frantic rushing around from one place to another can easily be seen in the form of muscle tension – hunched shoulders, tense necks, heads being constantly pulled back, strained and unhappy faces – and yet we do not begin life in this way.

George Orwell, the famous writer, once said that by the age of forty you get the face you deserve; perhaps the same could be said for the body. As young children we have all the time in the world, and consequently everything is of interest to us. This is reflected in the alertness of the eyes, the radiance of the face and the posture of the body. The seeds of the stress and tension that so many of us experience today are planted at an early age as part of the conditioning that takes place in modern society.

It seems rather curious that, thanks to modern technology, we have so many machines to make our lives easier – washing machines, dishwashers, cars, vacuum cleaners, computers, fax machines … the list goes on and on. In fact, during the late 1950s many people were seriously worried that they would have too much leisure time on their hands now that they had all these labour-saving devices! However, we actually seem to have far less time on our hands today, and many people feel under more and more pressure from a variety of sources. As a result, their quality of life – the very thing that they constantly wish to improve – is being severely affected.

Today, even a simple shopping trip can be a source of tension. We spend our precious time driving round and round looking for a parking space, and even when we find one there is usually a time limit imposed on us, so we rush around trying to get everything done before we get a parking fine. Many other activities, such as getting the children to school or arriving at work on time (or both!) can add to the stress, as the traffic on our roads becomes steadily worse. There is also increasing pressure, albeit subtle, imposed on both parents or partners to go out to work to improve the standard of living, yet the stress that this brings can often end in an unhappy family life

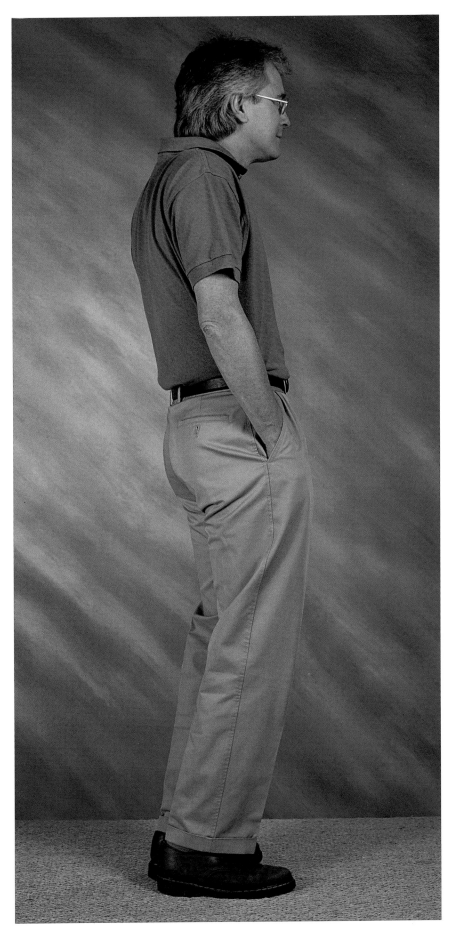

Left. *Many people have a faulty perception of themselves. This man thinks he is standing up straight when it is clear that he is leaning backwards from the waist. This causes his back muscles to contract and is likely to result in backache. It is often not until we catch ourselves in a mirror that we realize our movements are not at all as we intended.*

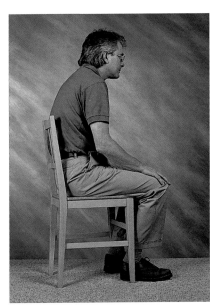

Above. *The 'fear reflex' (see page 29) causes muscle tension that can become habitually fixed within our body even when it is at rest. Notice how this man is raising his shoulders and how he is retracting his head back on to his spine. Over many years this posture has become his normal way of sitting, and it could contribute to a number of problems such as arthritis, general stiffness in old age, poor breathing and neck and back pain.*

with more and more arguments in the home. As a direct result of this pressure divorces have risen dramatically over the past twenty years, which is a clear reflection of the stress that many people are under. The results can be detrimental for both parents and children and the true damage may not be seen for generations to come.

It is important for us to realize that life is *not* an emergency just because many of us are acting as though it is. Although it may seem that there are not enough hours in the day to get everything done we really must give ourselves a chance to stop and think – if we continue to function under such pressure we are needlessly laying ourselves open to a number of stress-related ailments. Stress manifests itself in many ways. One is the fact that dentists are having to cope with an ever-increasing number of patients who, while sleeping or driving, are grinding their teeth together with an incredible amount of force. Their teeth become loose and, in time, fall out, and the surprising thing is that the patients themselves are completely unaware of the damage they are doing. Similar tensions can be seen throughout the body as muscles

pull bones together, causing unnecessary wear and tear on the bones and joints. It is these very tensions that the Alexander Technique can help us to ease or prevent.

True happiness

The Alexander Technique can help us to slow down and take each day as it comes, rather than trying to achieve more and more each day. We need to stop trying so hard and allow our lives to unfold naturally. To meet the deadlines, we are in fact wearing out our bodies more quickly than is necessary, as we deal with more stimuli than ever before. This is not helped by the fact that every day we are bombarded with advertisements which encourage us to believe that our lives are incomplete without a certain product: we begin to think that a particular car is going to give us the feeling of freedom that has been missing from our life; a certain toothpaste or shampoo will help us find that relationship we have always wanted; or a particular brand of beer is going bring us the happiness that has eluded us for years.

We all know, deep down, that we should not be living our lives in a state of dissatisfaction,

As this boy plays with his toy he is totally focused on what he is doing in that present moment. He is not thinking of all the things he would rather be doing, nor is he feeling guilty because he is enjoying himself. He is just being himself, experiencing a state of pure contentment which manifests itself as joy.

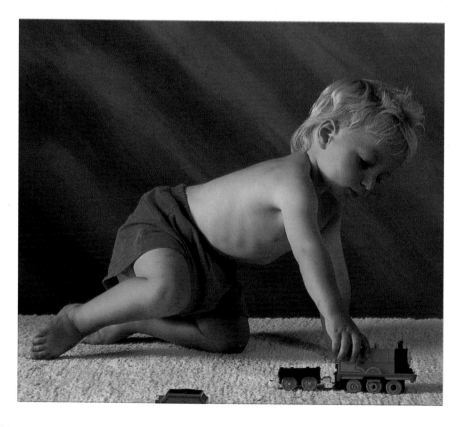

as this makes us feel that we continually have to strive to achieve a better lifestyle. The trouble is, the conditioning has been going on for longer than we can remember and the habits of the body, mind and emotions are so much a part of our lives that it is almost impossible to see another, easier way of being. We need to realize that the material possessions we are trying to acquire are not going to bring the happiness for which we long. Happiness comes from within: it is our birthright, something that all young children have naturally.

Alexander was absolutely convinced that his Technique could restore free choice to people's lives so that they could begin to live a more natural, harmonious life free from the tensions and worries that are so common today. In his book *Constructive Conscious Control of the Individual* he claimed that the lack of real happiness manifested by the majority of adults is due to the fact that they are experiencing a continually deteriorating use of their 'psycho-physical selves'. This deterioration is associated with certain character traits, flaws, temperament, and so on, characteristic of imperfectly co-ordinated people struggling through life beset with certain maladjustments. These maladjustments are actually setting up conditions of irritation and pressure during sleeping and waking hours. He went on to say that 'Whilst the maladjustments remain present, these malconditions increase day by day and week by week, and foster that unsatisfactory psycho-physical state which we call "unhappiness".'

The way we move is a mirror of our emotional state; when someone is in love, for example, you can see clearly that they begin to move in a very different way to their usual habits. Compare their movements to someone on the way to work, especially when it is a job they do not enjoy. It is easy to see the difference, but unfortunately peace of mind is becoming increasingly elusive and is being replaced with anxiety, unrest and a general lack of interest in the real things of life.

As we begin to grow away from our natural happy state of mind, fear begins to take over – fear of failure, ridicule, robbery, rejection and poverty, for example. As these fears begin to manifest in our lives, our muscles respond to them. We possess very powerful reflexes which come into operation when we are startled, a response that has come to be known as the 'fear reflex' (sometimes known as the 'fight or flight' startle pattern): the shoulders become hunched, the neck muscles tense, the chest flattens and the knees flex. This reflex is triggered in an emergency or when we are afraid, so that we are ready to act quickly, but in our day to day life it may come into operation when we are late for an appointment, under stress from work, or even when we become afraid of what the future holds. If these situations happen frequently enough, the tension in the neck and shoulders can become habitual, until we start to hold permanent stress in our bodies without realizing it *(see overleaf)*.

When I first started having Alexander lessons my teacher indicated that I had a lot of tension in my neck, of which I was completely unaware until one day when I was running late for an appointment. My route took me down a country lane, where I was delayed further by a herd of cows crossing the road. For a few seconds I could feel my chin protruding forward as my neck muscles contracted and my emotional fear reaction became stronger and stronger; I began to recognize just how much muscular tension I was exerting while merely sitting in the car performing no action whatsoever. It made me realize that it was actually my *mind* that was causing an emotional reaction, which in turn caused stress in my body.

End-gaining

Alexander firmly believed that most of our health problems occurred because as a race of people we had become totally goal-orientated. He referred to humans as a race of 'end-gainers', as we so often want to achieve an end without taking into consideration the means by which we achieve it. The very way in which we attempt to improve the quality of

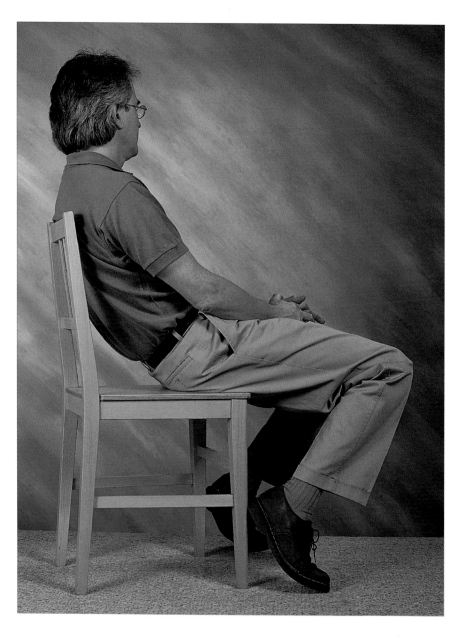

Many people misuse their body even when they are not performing activities – they become accustomed to sitting in a state of tension even when they think that they are relaxed. This man needs support from the back of the chair because his own postural muscles are no longer performing their supportive function. This is often due to the amount of time spent hunched over desks at work or at school – this alters our natural upright posture and we form bad habits that put our entire muscular system under strain.

our lives is not only wearing out our bodies at an accelerated rate, but could also be contributing to the destruction of the very planet on which we live. Alexander believed that unless we stopped and thought about the consequences of all our actions we would, in time, destroy ourselves on a global level in the same way we are destroying ourselves with muscular tension.

Practising the Alexander Technique teaches us to be aware of our actions, so that the choices we make are neither detrimental to ourselves nor our environment. Just consider some of the consequences of our end-gaining activities across the planet: man-made chemicals are responsible for damage to the ozone layer, causing an increase in levels of harmful ultraviolet radiation; the number of cars on the road increases every year, each one emitting carbon monoxide contributing to air pollution; vast areas of rainforest are destroyed every minute and at the current rate of destruction the rainforests may disappear altogether within the next hundred years, along with all the plant and animal species whose natural habitats they provide; and an estimated 10 million dolphins have been killed worldwide as a result of tuna fishing.

These are only a few examples of the irreversible damage we are doing to our world and there seems to be very little happening at present that will change the way we are living.

We are plundering our planet for our own immediate ends without a thought for future generations, and this attitude, whereby we strive to achieve our objectives without much concern for the consequences, carries through to our own bodies. We constantly place ourselves under stress and strain simply because we are so keen to realize our goals, regardless of what we do to ourselves in the process.

I remember watching an environmental programme on television as far back as 1970 called 'Owing to Lack of Interest Tomorrow Has Been Cancelled'. It outlined the dangers of pollution of the environment and called for immediate action to be taken by many leading scientists if we were to stand a reasonable chance of survival. Yet here we are, over a quarter of a century later, with pollution getting worse and worse by the day while everyone carries on apparently oblivious to the consequences. We have had one warning after another – how many more will there be before we decide to take constructive action that will bring about the changes that we so desperately need? Unless we can stop and take careful stock of how we live our lives, both individually and as a race of people, we could be heading for disaster. The same message has been given in many different ways, including this Native American saying:

Only when the last tree has died,
and the last river has been poisoned,
and the last fish has been caught,
will we realize that we cannot eat money.
[anon]

The Alexander Technique is not merely a way of improving posture and movement – it addresses every single issue that every human being faces during their life. Reason, choice and common sense are the supreme gifts with which all of us have been blessed, but unfortunately many of us do not use these qualities and instead we behave like lemmings, imitating the examples of others instead of thinking for ourselves. An interesting and humorous cartoon I saw recently depicted a queue of lemmings waiting to jump over a cliff, with the caption underneath, 'Two thousand lemmings can't be wrong'. Many of us just do as everyone else does, because as children we become afraid of being singled out, making a fool of ourselves or being ridiculed by our peer group. It takes an enormous amount of courage to think things through and then stand up for what you know in your heart to be right when faced with a variety of external pressures which encourage us to conform.

By following the principles of the Alexander Technique, which are set out in this book, we can become more conscious of the way we lead our lives; these principles will help us all to stop and *choose* the manner in which we wish to live. This can help in all aspects of our lives, from individual health problems to much wider issues such as benefiting our planet by being more conscious of our environment. There has never been a time when the physical, mental and emotional benefits of practising the Alexander Technique have been needed more. To discover where the stress starts in the first place, however, we need to look at the typical development of an 'educated' child.

The developing child

The way in which we are treated as children has an enormous effect on how we live our lives, and many of the behaviour patterns that we possess throughout our adult lives are formed in early childhood, or even as a young baby. Children learn everything they know from copying those around them, and at first they do not even judge the actions that they are copying. The habits of adults are copied unconsciously, often only emerging twenty or thirty years later.

Listening to an educational programme on the radio recently, I heard a school principal commenting that he was very concerned with the changes that he saw in children during their school years. He saw children of five or six start school with bright eyes, smiling faces, beautiful posture and ease of movement; they were nearly always talkative, eager to please, willing to learn and enthusiastic about life. By

31

the time these children left school they hardly looked anyone in the eye, their posture was very slumped with rounded shoulders, they were often lazy and uncaring about the people around them and they generally looked unhappy. 'What', he was asking, 'in the name of education are we doing to our children to make them change so dramatically?'

In my view the answer is simple: school, by its very nature, tends to remove children's freedom of choice. It does this physically by making them sit for long hours, mentally by putting them under stress at examination time,

and emotionally by making them feel out of place or foolish when they do not conform to the status quo.

At the age of four or five most children have beautiful posture; they move with great ease and agility. They are constantly varying their movements to suit their moods – sometimes hopping, then skipping, sometimes walking slowly and deliberately, and the next minute running wildly. They do not have to stress their bodies by being in certain places at definite times. Children of this age express themselves freely (text continues on page 36)

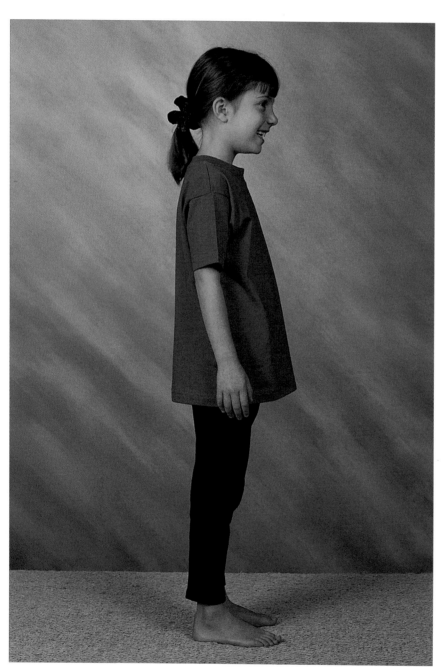

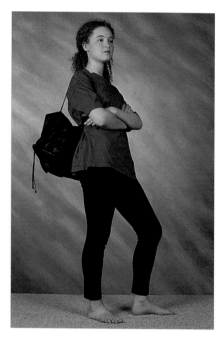

Left. *Young children have a natural spontaneity, and their posture is naturally 'perfect'. Notice how this six-year-old child is beautifully erect. This is often characteristic of children of this age, as they have not yet developed the bad habits that will gradually alter their posture.*

Above. *It is easy to see how the posture of a typical teenager is very different to that of a young child. Her heavy school bag is thrown over her right shoulder, which pulls her body out of balance and causes her to lean backwards and towards the right, with all her weight on her right leg. This misalignment places excessive strain on her spine and pelvic joint. Notice also the look of disinterest in her eyes.*

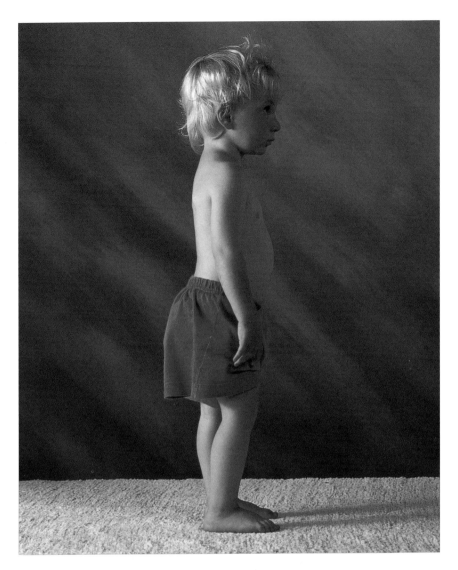

Left. *As children we naturally stand up straight – notice how this boy's head, spine, pelvis and legs are all in alignment. He is not 'doing' anything to achieve this – it is attained by his natural postural system which aligns his body without any physical effort on his part.*

Below. *The automatic reflex system controls every movement that we make. As the child's eyes see something to his right, his head turns the same way and the rest of his body follows a split second later.*

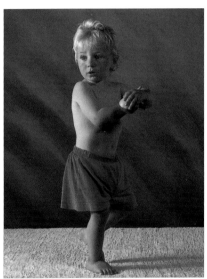

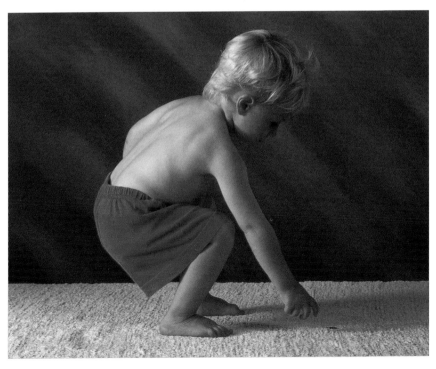

Left. *It is a joy to watch children move with grace and poise, which is achieved by the child being co-ordinated and balanced. Notice how this child has distributed his body-weight when bending down so that half of his weight is in front of his feet and the other half is behind. His head, neck and back are in a state of freedom, and this assists the free movement of his whole body.*

33

Right. *Even in a full squat the child maintains perfect balance effortlessly, and because there is no strain on the muscular system he can remain in this posture for as long as he needs to. In less industrialized countries, men and women squat like this throughout their entire lives.*

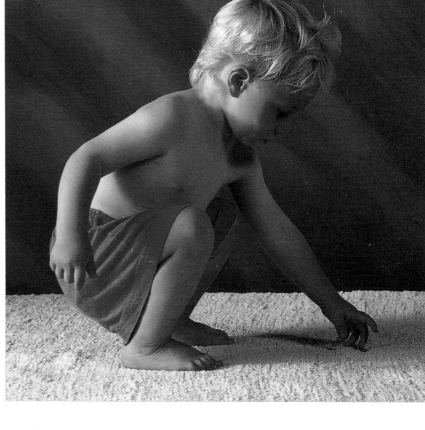

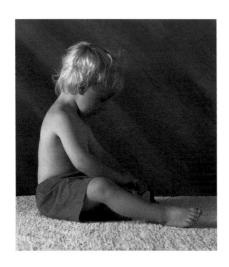

Above. *In all activities the child's posture is kept beautifully upright and the spine has a natural straightness that is unnecessarily lost as we grow older. You can see that although he is looking down he is not curving his back at all.*

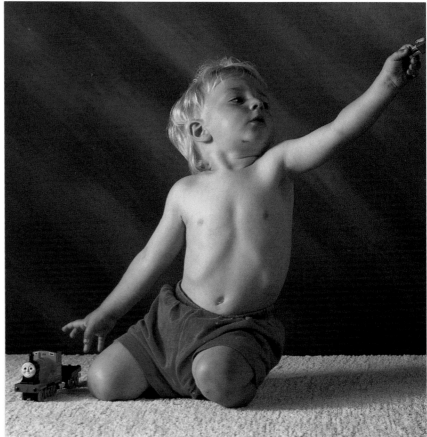

Right. *The boy reaches to full stretch with his left arm. His head and right arm automatically go the other way in order for him to keep his balance. He is totally absorbed ('present') in his action, unlike many distracted adults.*

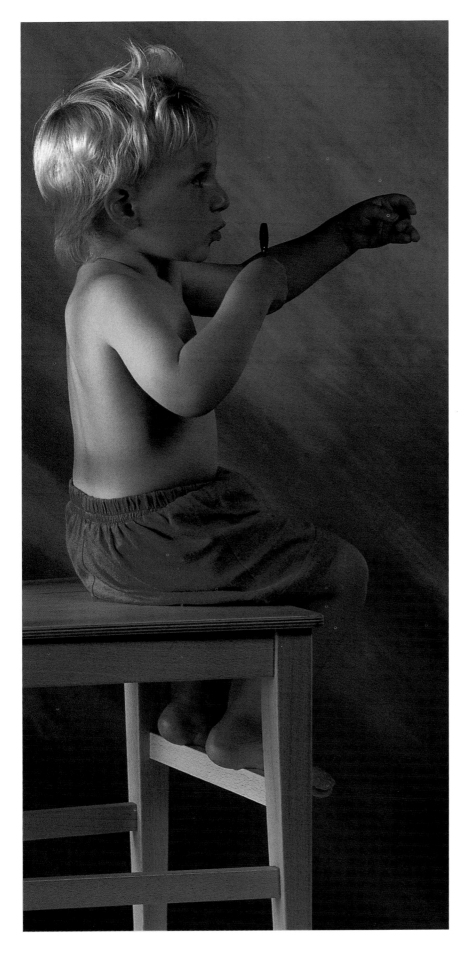

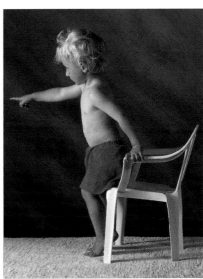

Left. *When sitting in a chair, young children hardly ever use the back of the chair for support – their postural reflexes allow them to sit supported and balanced for long periods of time without tiring.*

Above. *When a child moves, the head leads the movement and the rest of the body follows, with the result that the whole of the child's body is moving in one direction. This is often done with much enthusiasm and zest for life.*

and it is a pleasure to be near them; indeed, they are often thought of as having a free spirit.

In contrast, the natural maturation process causes most of this spontaneity to disappear, and by the time they leave school they have begun to adopt certain stereotypical movements which reflect the way they feel emotionally. For example, you can usually tell a teenager is shy or insecure simply by the way they hold themself – the lack of confidence tends to be reflected in a hunched posture, with the head hanging down so that eye contact can be avoided. These movements become ingrained and turn into unconscious habits, which frequently put disproportionate strains on certain muscles, joints and internal organs to the point where their bodies are no longer able to work efficiently; as adults we can usually recognize our friends merely by the way they stand or walk, and this is simply because of the particular habits they have developed over the years.

Often people think this is a normal part of getting old, but in unindustrialized societies the adults' posture and flexibility of movement remain unimpaired for most of their lives. In India or Africa, for example, the average sixty-year-old man or woman finds squatting easy and natural, which is not the case with most people in Western cultures.

Physical stress

At the age of five every child has to sit in a chair at school. Children tend to find school chairs rather uncomfortable as they are not really suited to their natural posture; this is largely because the seat of the chair, which takes most of the weight of the body, often

Right. *Nearly all young children hunch over their school work for many hours every day during the years when they are still growing and developing. Notice how the backward-sloping chair encourages this child to curve her spine instead of bending at the hip joint.*

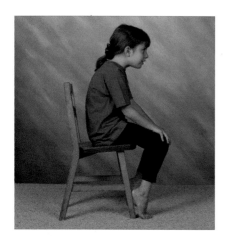

Above. *The slumped posture becomes a habit and the child will sit with a curved spine even when she is no longer sitting at her desk. This poor posture will squash the internal organs and adversely affect her breathing; the contracted state of her muscles physically pulls her body together and 'fixes' the rib-cage so that there is less room for her lungs to expand. The ribs should be in constant movement.*

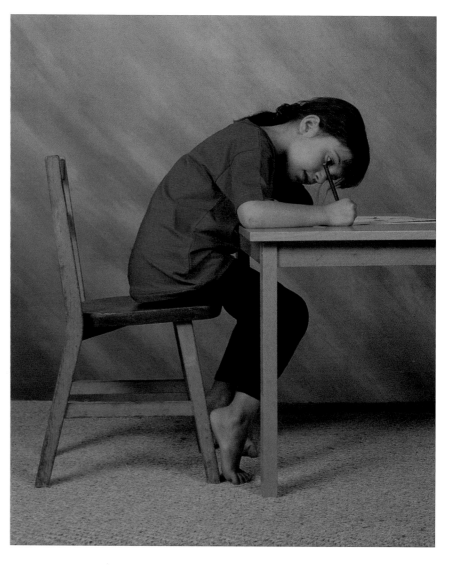

Right. *During Alexander lessons the child can be helped to be aware of her posture while writing at her desk and in other activities. Her back is now much straighter and her head is poised on top of her spine. This allows deeper breathing and will make her feel more alert. Her handwriting may even improve as her fingers relax; tension is often responsible for jerky movements.*

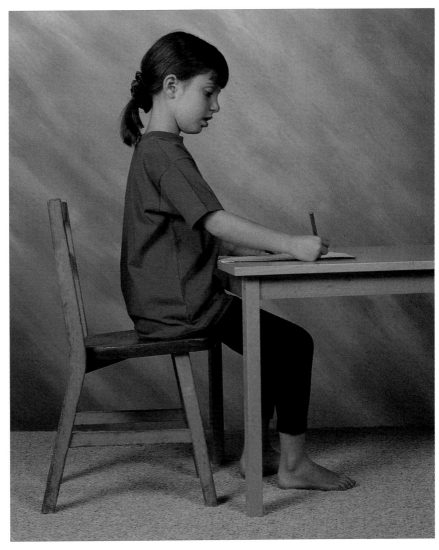

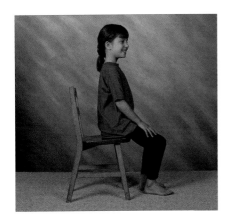

Above. *If the child is taught to maintain a balanced posture at her desk she is less likely to sit in a slumped manner at other times. This will affect her self-esteem and her general sense of well-being, and it will also help her to avoid adopting many bad habits that would affect her in later life.*

slopes backwards. This results in children having to tense many of their muscles to maintain the upright posture that is so natural to them when they are younger. They instinctively do not like this feeling at all and within minutes will often try to stand up or wander off. To combat the sense of 'falling backwards' that the chair produces, many children tilt forwards by raising the back legs of the chair off the floor, thus producing the effect of sitting on a forward-sloping chair. This position allows them to maintain their posture effortlessly.

Children have a natural ingenuity and intelligence which is why they instinctively try to maintain their natural posture as far as possible. Instead of asking *why* a child tilts the chair forward, an adult will usually tell the child exactly what they were taught when they were younger: 'don't swing on the chairs

– you will break them!' There is, of course, the danger that someone could trip over the back legs of the chair or that the child might tilt too far forward, and fall and become injured, but it is interesting that it is usually the damage to the chair that people give as a reason. The damage to the child's posture is not even considered at this stage, simply because most of us are unaware of the reason why children find so many chairs uncomfortable.

Children still do not give up; in their search for a comfortable position they often develop the technique of tucking one leg underneath them and sitting on it. This also has the effect of raising up the pelvis, once again enabling them to keep their upright posture. However, in most cases this is actively discouraged as it can interfere with the flow of blood down the leg. So, as children usually have to sit in

37

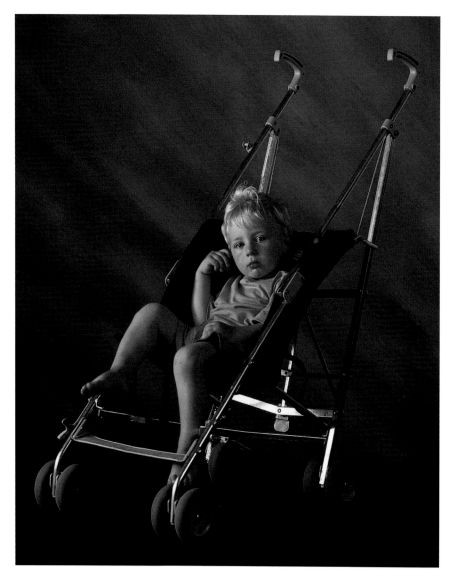

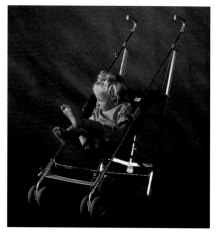

Left. *It is not only through sitting for long hours at school that the child's posture is affected. Many children's car seats and pushchairs encourage a slumped posture due to the fact that the seat tilts backwards, and this sows the seeds of poor posture in later life. This boy's postural muscles are not in use as he is being supported by the back of the chair. His head is not over his spine and his spine is not over his pelvis – he is totally out of alignment.*

Above. *A common sight is a child struggling hard to escape from the uncomfortable posture caused by the pushchair. Parents may often misinterpret this as naughty behaviour, but usually the child is simply trying to regain his or her natural poise.*

backward-sloping chairs for their whole school-life, sooner or later they will begin to slump as their back muscles become more and more fatigued. To make the problem worse, they then have to bend over their school work, and since it is difficult for them to use their hip joint (as the pelvis is already tilting backwards because of the shape of the seat), they will then bend their spine, causing unnecessary wear and tear on the vertebrae and discs.

This is a difficult problem to overcome. The best thing that parents can do is to be aware of the problem and make sure that the habits do not become too ingrained, although this can be tricky as children often ignore their parents' advice, especially if it makes them look like the odd one out at school. It might help for the child to sit on a wedge-shaped cushion at home *(see page 141 for details)* as this will encourage the body to revert to its natural posture for at least part of the day.

So, our children's posture deteriorates at school, largely through no fault of their own, and yet we blame them for having poor posture! They are told to sit up straight and put their shoulders back, and the only way to do this is to arch the lumbar spine with more tension than ever. They then begin to think that this is the way they ought to sit. Unfortunately, this posture becomes fixed within the body and can often remain throughout life, becoming progressively more painful as time goes on. These days the problem tends to start earlier than school because most children's pushchairs and car seats, which they use before they are one year old, are also sloping backwards *(see left)*. There are, however, a few that do not slope backwards and it is worth looking out for these; alternatively, parents could use sitting aids to help their child to maintain his or her natural posture *(see chapter four for more information on sitting)*.

Since many of us have been through this same process, it is hardly surprising that millions of people currently suffer with pain in the lumbar region. I am convinced that the posture we are told to hold as children and the phenomenal rise in back and neck pain in recent years are directly related.

Emotional stress

A large proportion of a child's development is spent in an environment of 'must', 'have to', 'can't', 'should', and 'ought to'. This has the detrimental effect of making children gradually lose their openness. Faced with their first days at school, many children scream, shout and have tantrums. Even the most loving parents leave their children crying at the school gate, probably against their natural feelings and parental instincts, because they believe this discipline is 'for the good of the child'. We should not forget that this is a very traumatic time for a child as it may well be the first major instance in which they feel abandoned and betrayed by their parents. Although parents can opt for private tuition for a child at home, the vast majority of children attend school. This means that most children have to learn to cope with being away from their parents in what is, at first, a totally unknown environment.

It is true that after a few weeks children 'settle down', but what is in fact happening is that they are learning how to conform to school life. School inevitably encourages us to act in a way that fits in with the rest of society – this is part of the educational process. However, we must not forget that, at first, children may find it hard to adapt to their new environment, and may even feel that their freedom has been taken away from them.

When my daughter was only four-and-a-half I was taking her along to her first day of school and she asked me, 'Daddy, how long do I have to go to school for?', to which I replied, 'You will finish this afternoon at four o'clock.' To my amazement she then said, 'No, no, I mean how many years do I have to go to school for?' It was then that I realized that some children see school as something they have to do from which there is no escape, and this must be a rather daunting prospect at such a young age!

For the vast majority of our early years some of us feel as though we are cooped up in an environment that is often confusing, humiliating and even at times hostile – especially for a five-year-old. We have to learn very quickly how to protect ourselves from punishment from teachers and ridicule and bullying from the other children. (I remember, as I know a great many other people also do, being ridiculed when giving a teacher the wrong answer to a particular question simply because I had misheard the question in the first place!) As a result, many children become more introverted and often think that there is something wrong with them, and this can give rise to a number of emotional problems in later life.

In the same vein, British principal Michael Sullivan wrote in an article in the *Times Educational Supplement* (18 October 1985):

> *'Self-confidence is developed through the reduction of fear, stress, uncertainty, confusion and failure – the very tools that too many of us skilfully use in the management of children in our charge. Children are fearful of verbal abuse, physical abuse and sarcasm. Children are stressed on the rack of tests and quizzes, often facing inevitable personal humiliation.'*

These are very strong words from a person who has worked in education for many years, but we hardly need to be told what we already know. Many of us have endured such traumas (some of us probably remember isolated incidents) but mostly we block out such memories because we would rather not think about them – yet our muscles remember them on an unconscious level. The protection that we acquire over those all-important years of our development manifests itself in muscle tension: our shoulders become rounded or hunched, our backs become arched and our stoops become more and more pronounced. These muscular tensions will subsequently affect the alignment of the rest of the body and can often be the seeds of future ill health. They will affect our lives on every level unless we are willing to release them from our body. Child psychologists can often detect children who are emotionally disturbed simply by the way they hold their body, which is often in a protective stance.

Mental stress

The educational system in most countries prepares children for a series of 'goal-orientated' examinations. They are encouraged to pass tests of increasing difficulty in order to qualify for entrance to colleges and universities to maximize their natural potential and hopefully seek employment in which they will be fulfilled and well paid. The money they earn will help them to have the freedom to be in control of their own lives.

The only trouble is that many people end up in jobs they dislike and yet have to work long hours, leaving very little time in which to do what they really want to do. Feeling dissatisfied, they look towards promotion, and an increase in salary, to fulfil themselves. They then find themselves trapped in a circle of ever longer hours and decreasing satisfaction, as they continually strive to achieve more, always looking for happiness in the future rather than in the present moment.

The constant pressure to perform under stressful conditions, whether at school or later on at work, is one of the primary causes of a

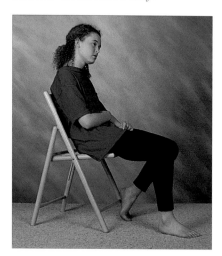

Below. *Even by the age of fifteen this girl's slumped posture has become her normal way of sitting. Many hours slumped over a desk have caused the muscles to shorten, distorting her natural upright posture. If this is allowed to continue it will cause excessive wear and tear on the entire body.*

Right. *After a few Alexander lessons this girl's posture has changed dramatically – her spine is much straighter and is now more able to perform its supportive function. The girl no longer feels that she has to use the back of the chair for support.*

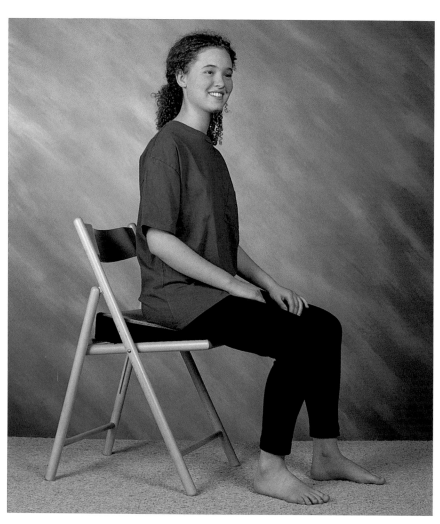

degenerating quality of life. Many people feel that something is missing from their lives, yet because many of us are in the same position we are not sure where to turn to increase our enjoyment, and often end up trying harder and harder, which is exactly the opposite of what we really need to do. When I was at school, practically every report I took home said, 'He must make more effort' or 'Could try harder' and this is what many people believe as they grow older; the harder they try, however, the further away they end up from the peace and contentment for which they long. In the end, our minds become so stressed that the small pockets of happiness we do experience become less and less frequent. Life is full of potential; we just need to stop long enough to appreciate the here and now, rather than hoping that things will get better in the future.

Self-confidence, which very young children possess naturally, can only be maintained by the absence of stress, confusion, uncertainty and, most of all, the fear of failure. Unfortunately, these are the very things many parents and teachers inflict on children in order to keep them under control. It is nobody's fault: it is often the only way adults know of dealing with children, for that is the way that they were treated as children themselves. How frequently do we tell our children how wonderful they are? Sadly, it is often the case that we are far too busy even to notice. Most of their 'naughty' behaviour patterns are only a desperate attempt to get noticed, as even the attention of an angry parent is better than no attention at all. Most of us will come across attention-seeking children at some point or other and you find that, instinctively, you try to ignore them.

Why we need the Alexander Technique

Through practising the Alexander Technique we can not only rid ourselves of physical tensions, but also free ourselves of many of the mental and emotional chains that we carry around which affect every decision and every movement we make. The Technique teaches us that we all have the freedom to choose what is best for us – we do not have to react in the habitual manner to which we have become accustomed. It shows us how to become more aware of our actions, so that we can react, both physically and mentally, in ways that are more appropriate to the situation. Simply by slowing down and taking the time to think about our actions we can learn how to use our bodies better, in order to avoid the many aches and pains that are often thought of as age-related. If we are able to recognize and let go of tension we will be able to achieve a more relaxed physical state. This will be reflected in our mental attitude and should help us to become calmer and happier as we go about our daily activities. This book will soon show you how to apply the principles of the Alexander Technique to your life, and how to begin to reclaim the natural poise and spontaneity that we each possess as a child.

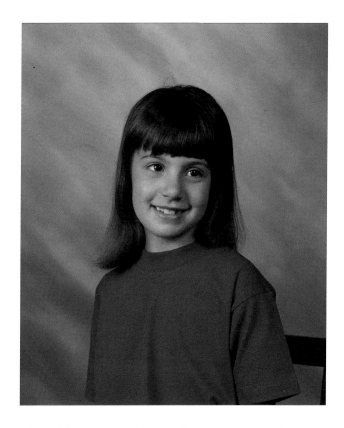

The child's face is a reflection of an inner tranquillity – sheer enjoyment of being in the present moment. This quality is later eroded by all the stresses and strains of living at such a fast pace. In less industrialized countries, where the pace of life is much slower, the serene quality in people's faces often remains present throughout their lives.

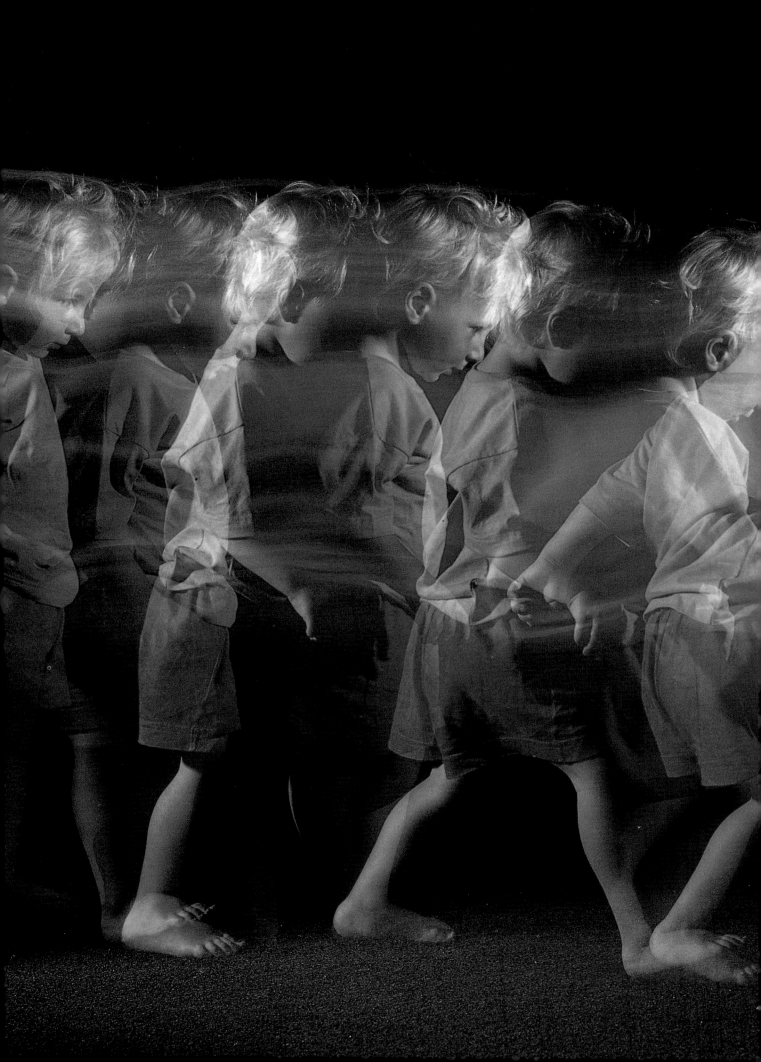

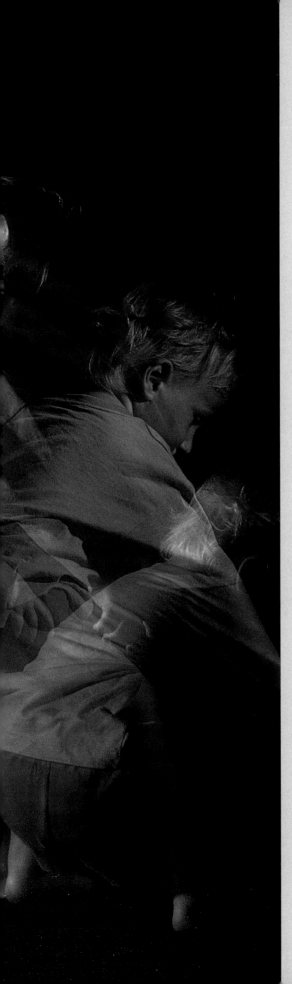

CHAPTER THREE

Pausing
before action

'At the still point of the turning world.
Neither flesh nor fleshless;
Neither from nor towards;
At the still point, there the dance is,
But neither arrest nor movement.
And do not call it fixity.
Where past and future are gathered.
Neither movement from nor towards,
Neither ascent nor decline.
Except for the point, the still point,
There would be no dance,
And there is only the dance.'

T. S. Eliot

Before we can change any of our habitual ways of
moving we first have to pause and consciously choose
a different way of moving. In children this process of
inhibition is instinctive – this child automatically squats
down to pick something up rather than bending from the
waist – but as we get older we lose this ability. Learning
to inhibit is a vital aspect of the Alexander Technique.

Pausing before action

Inhibition is one of the fundamental principles behind the Alexander Technique and, without it, it is impossible for us to change any of our habits even once we have recognized them. Inhibition is simply when we pause first before reacting instinctively in any given situation. Many people associate inhibition with the suppression of feelings or the inability to be spontaneous, but this is mainly because the famous psychologist Sigmund Freud used the term in this negative context. The actual dictionary definition of inhibition is: *the restraint of direct expression of an instinct.*

If the restraint is done unconsciously out of fear due to past experiences, then it could be seen as having negative connotations. However, if the mental act of inhibition is done consciously and for a particular reason then the result can have great advantages for the way in which we behave, and we can gain greater control by actively choosing what we do or do not want to do in our lives. For people who practise the Alexander Technique, inhibition has a very definite purpose: it helps us to stop reacting in a stereotyped manner so that our true spontaneity can emerge, and it does this by delaying the instantaneous and conditioned responses that we have learned throughout our lives.

Two hundred years ago life was far more simple, but today there are numerous stimuli that bombard our senses each day. Just walk down a busy street in any town or city and observe how much noise and visual movement we have to cope with all the time. We do this without giving it a second thought, yet we often feel tired afterwards because our nervous system has been under excessive strain. A moment of pausing gives us the opportunity to act with greater consciousness, providing a chance to act in a manner that is more appropriate to the situation, rather than unconsciously reacting with unnecessary muscular tension.

Why do we need to inhibit?

Inhibition helps to prevent any interference with the primary control (the relationship of the head, neck and back). If our body is to remain in a state of freedom and our posture is to be balanced, it is essential that the head remains in a poised state on top of the spine. In stressful situations our 'fear reflex' is triggered: this causes us to hunch our shoulders and pull our head back and downward on to our spine. If we are under constant stress at work, at school or at home the primary control is continually being interfered with, and eventually this tension in the neck muscles becomes a habit that occurs even when we are not under pressure. This interference is transmitted to other muscles throughout the body, producing a lack of balance and co-ordination and often resulting in excessive muscular tension, causing the body to wear out before its time.

Inhibition is not only helpful when carrying out actions such as walking and bending, but is also useful when reacting emotionally during arguments, for example. If we are able to pause and calmly put across our point of view, then we are much more likely to be able to achieve our desired result. It can be instrumental in changing the way we live, on both an individual and a global level.

Natural inhibition

In animals inhibition is instinctive; just observe a domestic cat for a few minutes and you will see it pause just before many of its movements. The more important the activity is to the cat, the longer the cat will wait so it can get the timing exactly right, and by doing so it can judge the length of a leap with remarkable accuracy *(see page 46).*

Observing animals in their natural habitat, Alexander wrote: 'The wild cat stalking its quarry inhibits the desire to spring prematurely,

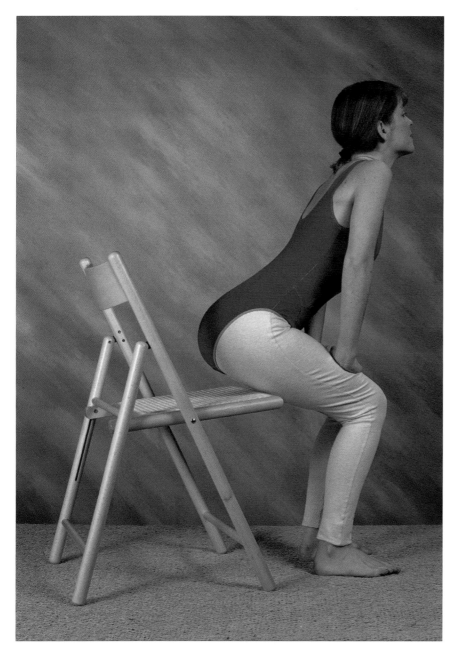

Left. *Notice that this woman is getting out of her chair with far more effort than is really necessary. Even before she has left the chair, her head is retracting backwards, causing a shortening of the entire spine; as a result, the intervertebral discs are squashed and this could possibly contribute to the problem of slipped discs in the long run. She is also preparing to lever herself up by pushing down on her thighs, making the leg muscles work much harder than they need to.*

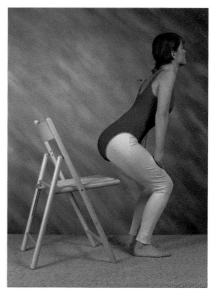

Right. *You can see how her shoulders hunch and her neck muscles tense as she pulls her head back. This is the same reaction as if she had been frightened, which means that she has acquired a habit of moving with her 'fear reflex' in operation.*

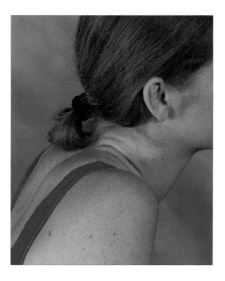

Above. *Throughout the movement her back is arched, and this is caused by over-tightened back muscles. If these muscles are constantly over-strained, as is often the case, the result can be damage to the intervertebral discs. She could also find that she suffers from neck pain, as a result of chronic wear and tear from frequent compression of the vertebrae in the neck.*

45

and controls to a deliberate end its eagerness for the instant gratification of a natural appetite.' Inhibition is sometimes mistakenly interpreted as performing actions slowly, but if we look again at the cat family we find that, although natural inhibition is prevalent, they are among the fastest creatures on earth.

Small children also inhibit many of their movements and they are not afraid to say 'no' to many of the demands that are placed on them – in fact, it is often their favourite word. Frequently you see them deliberately pausing before answering questions or performing actions. This natural inhibition tends to disappear as we grow older.

It is the same with adults in unindustrialized societies – we often consider the African women carrying water on their heads as having good posture as they walk with grace and poise, but if you notice how they move you will also see that they are never in a hurry and do not have the same concept of time as many people in Western society. In fact, very few of them even own a watch. In industrialized societies, by contrast, people often rush into situations without thinking about the consequences, frequently making mistakes that could have been avoided. We even become irritated when the people in front of us in a queue or on the roads seem to be taking their time. We are often so totally goal-orientated that we hardly ever give thought to the way in which we perform activities; we do not even see why it is important to consider our actions, as long as the job gets done.

Conscious inhibition

Unless we can learn how to pause before acting and bring our thoughts away from past and future matters, so we can attend to the way we go about our lives, we will not be able to avoid many of the health problems that plague us in later life. In numerous cases, it is not until people are in extreme pain that they will give even a minute's thought to how they move. Our body is our most precious possession, and yet most of us look after our cars better than we do ourselves. It is vital that we learn how to look after our bodies if we want them to work well and be pain-free in later life.

When a cat is stalking its prey, it always pauses (inhibits) before moving, waiting for the right moment before it pounces. This act of inhibiting gives the cat the highest chance of success. Inhibiting is not about performing actions slowly – after all, cats are among the quickest animals on earth.

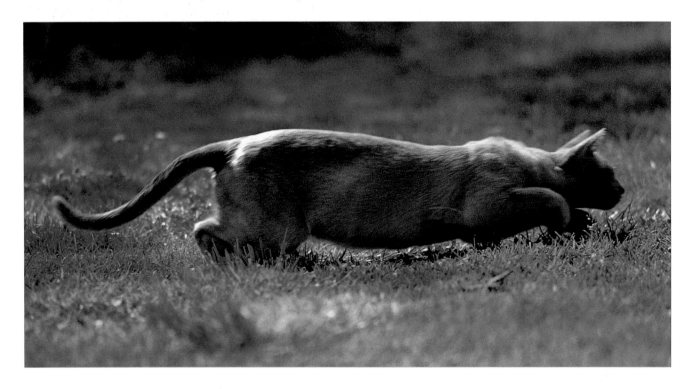

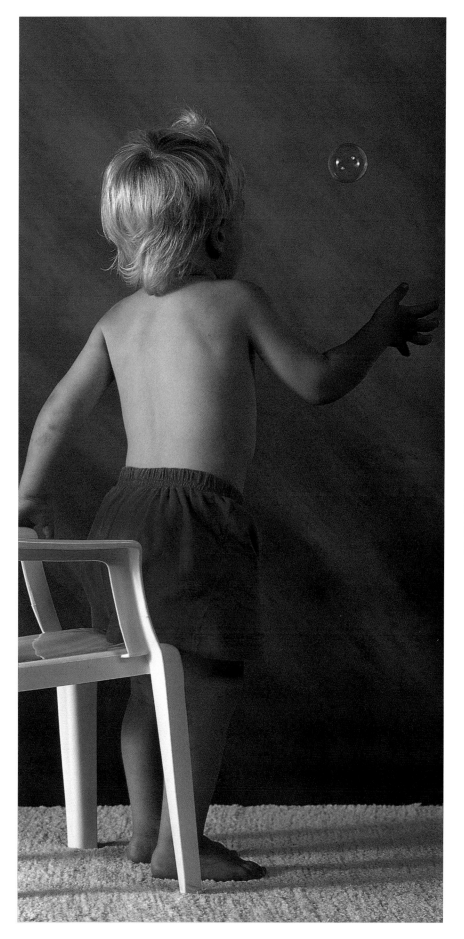

Below. *The child's natural inhibition can be easily seen as he pauses and waits for the bubble to land on his hand. He is totally still and only aware of what is happening in that moment.*

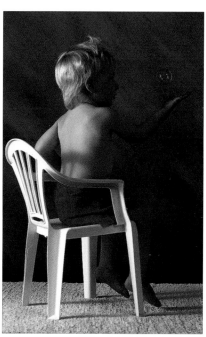

Left. *As the bubble moves away from his hand, the child follows it with his eyes and his head naturally moves towards the object of interest. As his head leads this movement, the rest of his body will spontaneously follow with grace and ease.*

In his best-selling book, *The Ascent of Man*, Dr Jacob Bronowski wrote: 'We are nature's unique experiment to make the rational intelligence prove sounder than the reflex.' He then went on to say that the success or failure of this experiment depends on our ability to impose a delay between the stimulus and our response. In other words, unless we are able to learn consciously to inhibit before acting, we will probably be heading for the extinction of our own species. We are creatures who have evolved away from our primitive instincts and as yet have no tools with which to replace them. Conscious inhibition is just such a tool.

I find that the most difficult aspect of the Alexander Technique which many people find hardest to put into practice is the ability to pause before they act. They feel that they hardly have time to think and often feel under pressure to perform a number of activities in a limited amount of time. The concept of stopping for a second or two before they move seems, to them, a pure indulgence.

As the pace of life increases, it actually becomes even more important to slow down and take your time when making decisions. Is it not strange that there is rarely enough time to do a job properly in the first place, but there is *always* enough time to go back and correct the mistakes? The fact is that there is as much time as we allow ourselves. The clock is a tool that we use for our convenience, yet somehow we end up becoming a slave to time. In my ex-perience, the feeling that there is not enough time in the day probably causes more muscular tension in modern society than anything else.

The act of inhibiting has an immediate calming effect on the entire skeletal, respiratory, nervous and muscular systems: our breathing becomes slower and deeper; our muscles are more relaxed; our nervous system does not have to cope with over-stimulation; and our skeletal system is under less strain. This gives us enough time to act with both ease and free choice. Inhibition is not a static or passive process but is an act in itself, employing the entire nervous system. Next time you see a domestic cat pausing before chasing a bird, mouse or even a piece of string, notice that although the cat's head will be very still, its hind legs will be preparing for the movement. Alexander saw inhibition not as suppression, but as volition. It enables us to do what we have decided we want to do.

Inhibition can also be very important with regard to breathing. If we react quickly we are likely to interfere with our breathing pattern, taking short, shallow breaths, and in some cases we may even hold our breath altogether. When we pause before acting we feel that we have more time, and our breathing tends to be deeper and less rushed, allowing its natural cycle to take place. Natural respiration is essential for physical, emotional and mental well-being.

Freedom of choice is the main characteristic that sets us apart from the rest of the animal kingdom, supposedly making us 'the crown of creation'. Animals follow their instincts, yet we have the ability to think, reason and, if necessary, override these instincts if we think it is more advantageous to do so. In other words, if a cat were being chased by a dog, it might well run across a road and be killed in its endeavour to escape from its predator; it follows its instinct to run from immediate danger. Humans, on the other hand, can stop and choose the best course of action to take, even if it means going against our basic instincts.

If our freedom to choose were threatened by another nation we would risk life and limb to preserve the privilege of free choice; that is how important it is to us. Yet many of us do everything out of habit alone, giving little thought to how we move or how we think and rarely exercising our freedom to choose. Many people think that the Alexander Technique is about performing certain actions in a particular way – that there are right ways and wrong ways of doing things. This is definitely not the case, for it goes much deeper than this: it goes to the very core of human existence and also to the heart of the whole question of human evolution and the future of the human race. The Alexander Technique

THE BENEFITS OF INHIBITION

The benefits of applying inhibition before acting are enormous; it can transform the way you live. As a result you will feel much more in control of your life, and this will automatically lead to a happier and a more fulfilling existence. The ways that inhibition can benefit you are as follows:

- *It gives you more time to think of the most appropriate way of performing actions.*
- *It helps you to prevent over-tensing your muscles, allowing your natural reflexes to co-ordinate and balance your body with ease.*
- *It gives you time to be aware of any stress you may be putting on any part of your body.*
- *It helps you to be more aware of your habits and allows you to change them if you so wish.*
- *It gives you a chance to say 'no' to taking on projects that will put you under stress.*
- *It gives you a chance to apply your directions before you act (see chapter four).*
- *It can save you time, because you are less likely to make mistakes which take time to correct.*
- *It encourages deeper, calmer breathing patterns.*

gives you a choice about how you treat not only yourself, but also your environment. Alexander himself once clarified his Technique in the following way:

'Boiled down, it all comes to inhibiting a particular reaction to a given stimulus. But no one will see it that way. They will see it as getting in and out of a chair the right way. It is nothing of the kind. It is that a pupil decides what he will or will not consent to do.'

Without inhibition there can be no change; our habits will always prevail, and if we do what we have always done we will obviously get the same results that we always have. Generally, people tend to harbour a fear of the unknown and are very resistant to any change in their lives – I often find that although people who come to me actually want change because of some physical or emotional pain, they still want their lives to remain essentially the same. We need to overcome this fear if we are to help ourselves in the long term.

It is an interesting thought that we now own cars that can accelerate from 0 to 60 mph in a matter of seconds and are capable of reaching speeds in excess of 100 mph, but we never ask ourselves, 'Where am I heading for, and why do I need to get to my destination so quickly?' It is important to pause frequently and ask, 'What is it I really want to achieve in my life, and am I going in the right direction to attain those goals?' It is time for us to think about our *actions*, rather than just being concerned with what our actions can achieve.

As the pace of life becomes more frantic by the year, the ability to pause and choose becomes even more essential if we are to survive the ever-increasing pressure, most of which is self-inflicted. When the elements of speed, competition and goal-orientation are removed from an activity, great pleasure can be found in the simplest of tasks. Anyone can consciously inhibit before acting – all it takes is determination and a realization of how important it is to our well-being.

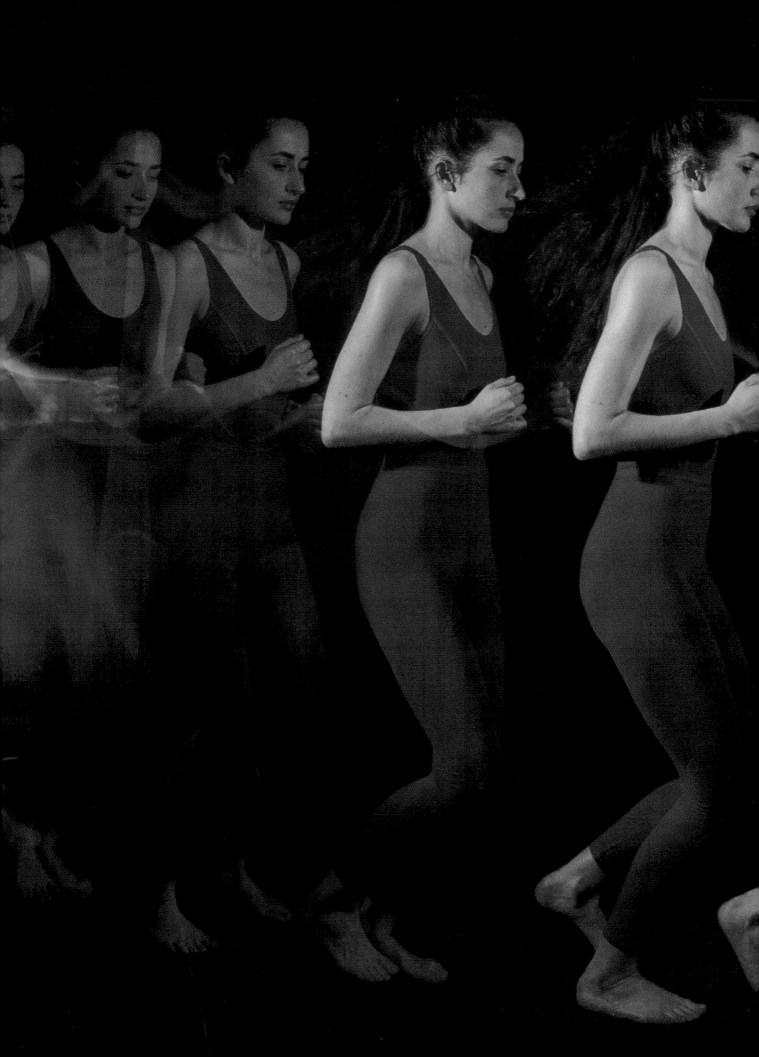

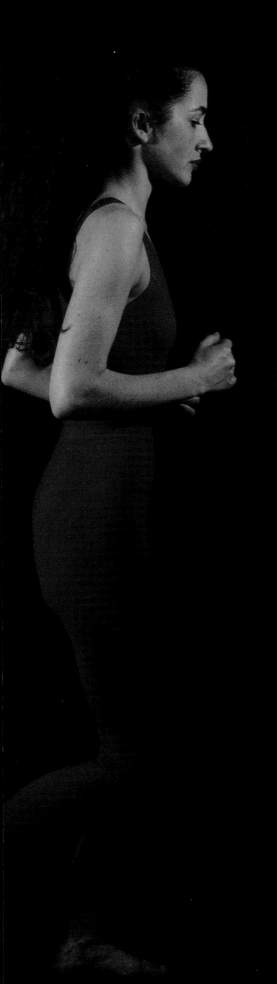

CHAPTER FOUR

Thinking in activity

*'People travel to wonder at the heights
of mountains, at the huge waves of the sea,
at the long courses of rivers, at the vast
compass of the ocean, at the circular
motion of the stars; and they pass by
themselves without wondering.'*

Saint Augustine

*By being aware of tension and releasing it, you will be able
to use your body much more efficiently. Alexander devised a
unique system of 'directions' which involves using the power of
the mind to release physical tension. This woman is applying
her directions as she runs, and as a result her body is in
alignment and she is moving freely and easily.*

Thinking in activity

Thoughts are powerful. The way in which we think determines, to a great extent, the path of our lives. There was a case in Taunton, England, in 1974, of a woman who was suing the National Health Service for giving her the wrong medical information. She was told incorrectly that she was suffering from an incurable form of cancer; she actually lost 38 kg (6 st) and her body exhibited all the relevant symptoms. Eventually she was admitted to a hospice and everyone, including herself, thought she was terminally ill. It was at this point that she was informed that they had mixed up the X-rays and that there was, in fact, nothing wrong with her at all, and as a result her health immediately began to improve. This is a clear demonstration of the connection that our mind has with our body and emotions.

If a child is brought up to believe that life is difficult and everything is a struggle, then that is probably what it will turn out to be. Similarly, if a child is taught that life is a pleasure, then the chances are that they will have a joyful and optimistic life. There is an old saying that if you bring half a glass of water to an optimist, and then to a pessimist, they will each have a different reaction; the optimist will be very grateful and quench his thirst eagerly while the pessimist will start complaining that the glass is only half full.

Alexander discovered that his mind had a powerful effect on his body, and, while he was trying harder and harder to recite, he was creating a build-up of tension in his neck muscles which affected his entire body.

He also found out that he could order his body to release that tension, and he referred to this procedure as 'directing' the body. Directions are mental orders that you give to yourself to prevent unnecessary muscular tension occurring during any activity that you perform during the course of your day. To many people it may seem like a strange usage of the word, but in the world of stage and performance it is not uncommon to be aware of the way you are directing yourself.

Giving directions

In Alexander terms, to give a direction is: *a process which involves projecting messages from the brain to the body's mechanisms, and conducting the energy necessary for the use of these mechanisms.*

Tension invariably causes the muscles to shorten; in contrast, directions involve thinking of different parts of the body lengthening or widening away from one another, resulting in the easing of any unnecessary tension. With directions, you can release any part of the body from any other part of the body – the two areas do not necessarily have to be directly connected. People often think of the Alexander Technique as a way of relaxing, but although their body does become less tense or rigid this does not mean that they allow their limbs to go completely slack or limp.

By becoming aware of tension throughout the body in all our activities, and using the tools of inhibition and direction, we can bring our bodies back into a natural state of balance. This allows the entire muscular system to work in harmony, instead of forcing the muscles to work against each other, as is often the case. It is obvious that we do need a certain degree of muscle tone in order to perform any action; what the Alexander Technique helps us to do is to have the appropriate muscle tone for the activity we are performing.

All your mechanisms and reflexes are designed to help your body to lengthen, and by applying directions you can get in touch with habits that prevent this from happening; when you release tension, your body will automatically lengthen and widen. Some people tend to concentrate in a very purposeful and serious manner when they are giving themselves the directions, but this is more likely to result in an increase of tension, achieving the opposite of what they intended. In my view, directions are gentle thoughts, more like wishes than determined or goal-orientated thoughts. When talking about posture, Alexander once said that there was no such thing as a right position, but there was such a thing as a right direction.

Directions are split into two categories: *primary* and *secondary*. Each category has a different function, depending on exactly where in the body you want to release tension.

Primary directions

Most of the problems that stem from poor posture can be traced to over-tensed neck muscles that interfere with the freedom of the head in relationship to the spine. If this freedom is not present it is impossible to obtain any lasting freedom elsewhere in the body. Alexander referred to the relationship between the head, neck and back as the 'primary control' and discovered that it governed the workings of all the body's mechanisms, thus making control of the complex human being relatively simple.

Freedom of movement requires that the primary control be allowed to work without any restriction (it is likely that Alexander only made this discovery because his voice problem was caused by tension in the neck muscles). The main directions allow the primary control to return to its natural state of freedom, and consequently affect reflexes and muscle tension throughout the body.

THE PRIMARY DIRECTIONS

1. Think of allowing your neck to be free.
2. Allow your head to go forward and up.
3. Allow your back to lengthen and widen.

It is important that the directions are given in this sequence, as you cannot obtain satisfactory results if the preceding direction has not been carried out. In other words, it is impossible to allow the head to go forward and up if you have not released the tension in the neck, and, similarly, it is impossible to achieve a lengthening in the spine if the head is not going forward and up.

Think of allowing your neck to be free

The aim of this instruction is to release any excessive tension that may exist in the neck area resulting in the head being pulled backwards. The place to put our awareness is at the top of the spine and base of the skull, which is much higher at the back than it is at the front. It is important to realize that tension in the neck is often hard to perceive, because there are fewer tension-detecting receptors in the neck muscles than in other parts of the body. It also follows that even when you have applied this direction you may not be aware of the tension you have released. It is vital that you only use your thoughts when applying this direction, rather than physically moving your head, as this will only increase the muscular tension.

Allow your head to go forward and up

The head goes forward and up in relation to your spine and *not* in relation to your environment. Most of our senses are in the head, and because of this the body is organized in such a way that the head leads and the body follows. Allowing the head to go forward helps a natural organization to occur, permitting any movement to be done with the maximum efficiency. If we only allow the head to go forward there is a danger of it drooping, and to counteract this it is important to think of the head going upwards as well.

Allow your back to lengthen and widen

This direction will help you to release tension throughout the upper part of your body. Expanding this area will improve your breathing and allow all the internal organs more space, enabling them to function more efficiently. It will also prevent a shortening of the spine, which can often cause or aggravate back and neck pain. Releasing tension in the upper part of your body will also ease the downward pressure that can cause unnecessary restriction in the movement of the hips, legs and feet, which makes standing and walking more difficult.

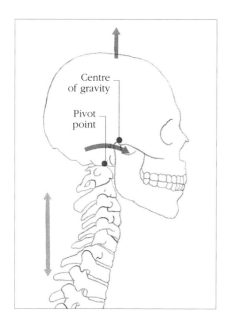

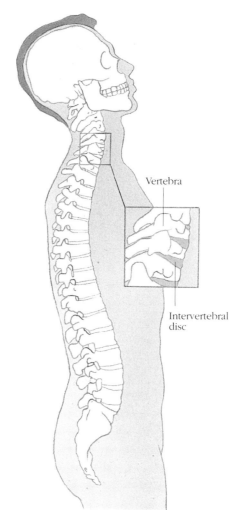

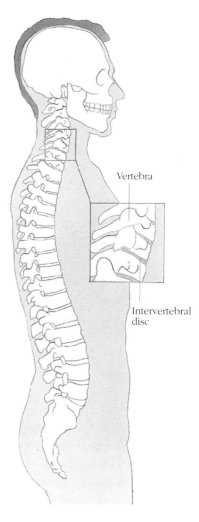

The arrows illustrate the primary directions – the mental directions that you need to give yourself before you can release tension in any other area of the body.

● Allow your neck to be free. *You need to direct your thoughts to the pivot point located at the top of the spine in order to release tension in the neck.*

● Allow your head to go forward and up. *This encourages the body to work as nature intended. It is important to get your Alexander teacher to show you how to apply these directions.*

● Allow your back to lengthen and widen. *This encourages your spine to elongate rather than to shorten, and causes movement without any excessive muscular effort.*

When the head is retracted the vertebrae in the neck are forced back on to each other and the whole spine becomes shortened. This crushes the intervertebral discs and, if done habitually, may cause neck or spinal problems.

When the head is poised on the top of the spine it allows the spine to lengthen; the vertebrae are equally spaced due to minimal muscular tension. This means that neck and back problems are likely to be avoided.

Secondary directions

These are a supplement to the main directions and can be used to release tension in localized areas of the body, but they do not affect the functioning of the primary control as much as the primary directions. Remember that you must always apply your primary directions *before* applying any secondary ones. The following directions are some of the ones that you will find most useful:

● *Allow your shoulders to release away from one another.* This will help a release across the upper chest area and is very beneficial to anyone who has rounded shoulders.

● *Allow your left shoulder to release away from your right hip, and your right shoulder to release away from your left hip.* It is very common for people to pull down with their front muscles; leaning over a school or office desk for many years is often the reason. This direction can help us to free the tension that this habit encourages.

● *Allow your hands to lengthen away from your shoulders.* This will help you to let go of any tension in your arms and can be particularly useful for those who have a habit of hunching their shoulders.

• *Think of allowing your hands to widen as your fingers lengthen.* This can help anyone who clenches their fists unconsciously when under stress.

• *Think of not pushing your pelvis forward.* This can prevent an over-arching of the back and the common habit of leaning backwards when standing.

• *Think of not bracing your knees back.* This can be effective in the release of tension in the legs. Be careful that you do not start to over-compensate by standing with your knees bent.

• *Think of your feet spreading on to the ground as your toes lengthen.* This can release tension in the feet, which is often the cause of common foot problems. It will also help you to feel more balanced.

• *Think of your lower jaw releasing from your ears.* This helps to eliminate excessive tension in the facial muscles, which is very common.

These are only a few of many secondary directions, but they all entail allowing one part of your body to release away from another part. In addition, you can also direct your whole body in a certain direction; when the head leads a movement, the rest of the body naturally follows in the same direction as a result of the body's natural reflexes.

COMMON PITFALLS

There are a number of things that people tend to do wrong when they start giving themselves directions. Here are just a few things to watch out for:

• *People tend to actively 'do' the directions instead of merely thinking of them. This usually results in increasing muscle tension rather than reducing it.*
• *People often become impatient when they do not 'feel' anything happening and may give up. They do not realize that their muscles are in fact releasing without their conscious knowledge.*
• *The directions need to be practised over and over again, until the student is completely familiar with them. It is only then that the directions will be stronger than the student's old habits. It is exactly the same as when learning to play a musical instrument or learning to drive, for example: you have to spend hours and hours practising.*

Breathing

Breath is the essence of life; the first thing you do when you enter this world is breathe, and it is the last thing you do when you leave. Everyone knows that breathing is the most fundamental requirement of the human body and that without it we cannot survive for more than a few minutes, yet most of us give it very little attention. In fact, not only do we breathe to survive, but our health and general well-being depend on the *way* we breathe, and it is therefore vital that we relearn how to breathe naturally.

If you observe a baby or young child you will see that the abdomen moves in and out rhythmically with each breath, while the upper chest and shoulders remain in a state of relaxation and are relatively still. Yet in many adults the opposite happens; the abdomen remains rigid, forcing the rib-cage to be pushed up on the in-breath and then to collapse on the out-breath. I find that when people first

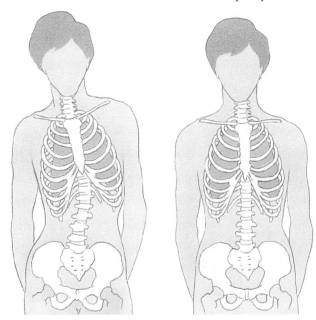

Muscular tension can cause your frame to be twisted or pulled over to one side, and can result in one or both of the lungs having less room to move (above left). Shallow breathing is the inevitable result: it causes stale air to occupy more of the lungs, and so the lungs become less efficient in expelling waste products. Breathing then becomes faster, which can give rise to anxiety, as the body is not taking in as much oxygen as it needs. If we allow our postural muscles to support us naturally, our frame will be upright and our lungs will have sufficient room in which to function properly (above right).

come for lessons their breathing is often very erratic or too fast; they do not even give themselves time to finish one breath before they start the next. This is a direct reflection of how they are living their lives – at a fast pace with never enough time to get everything done. The stress that many people are under causes excessive muscular tension, restricts their breathing and results in breathing habits, such as shallow breathing, fast breathing and little movement of the diaphragm and ribs, that are detrimental not only to their bodily functions, but also their state of mind and quality of life.

The first thing to do to improve your breathing is simply to become aware of your breath without trying to change it. Just by placing your attention on how you breathe will bring about an improvement by encouraging you to take longer and deeper breaths. Contrary to what many people think, it is the out-breath that controls the way we breathe, because it causes a vacuum in our lungs which allows the next inhalation to be taken spontaneously and without effort. To help his students relearn how to breathe naturally, Alexander developed the following procedure, which is known as 'the whispered ah'.

THE WHISPERED AH

Regular practice of this technique will help you to notice detrimental breathing habits and will lead to a more efficient respiratory system. It will help you to realize how deeply you can breathe, and how you have only been using a fraction of your lung capacity.

- *First notice where your tongue is and let it rest with the tip lightly touching the lower front teeth.*
- *Make sure your lips and facial muscles are not tensed. You may find it helpful to think of something amusing.*
- *After you finish your next in-breath, open your mouth by letting your jaw drop (make sure your head does not tilt backwards in the process).*
- *Whisper an 'ah' sound until you come to the natural end of the out-breath.*
- *Gently close your lips and allow the air to come in through your nose and fill up your lungs.*
- *Repeat several times.*

Discovering and releasing tension

As you become more familiar with the tools of inhibition and direction you will begin to become more aware of areas of tension in your body that you have perhaps never considered before. Here are some everyday activities that demonstrate exactly why we need to 'think in activity' – so that we can become aware of our habits and make conscious choices to benefit ourselves.

Standing

Even when we are standing still our body is performing a miraculous balancing act. The reflexes in the body organize the extremely unstable structure of our bones, muscles and organs into an upright posture without any thought on our part. In every muscle there are postural and activity muscle fibres. The activity muscle fibres are for movement and are activated consciously, whereas the postural muscle fibres keep you upright and are activated subconsciously by the body's reflexes.

If you look around you in a busy street, however, you will often find people leaning backwards or leaning forwards while they are standing, with their weight over to one side, or even supported by only one leg. Most of them will be completely unaware that they are standing in such awkward ways, or that the positions they have adopted may cause posture-related problems in later life. Even when we make the effort to improve our posture by 'standing up straight' we often arch our backs and lean backwards, which quickly leads to a feeling of tiredness, and once again we feel the need for external support (*see opposite*). In turn, this can often lead to a feeling of being unsupported emotionally. Using the Alexander Technique we can re-educate our entire muscular system so that our postural muscles support us naturally. By giving directions we can release the tension in our muscles so that the postural muscles, which do not tire so easily, can do their job of keeping us upright. Usually, we hold ourselves up by our activity muscle fibres, which tire quickly; this is what gives rise to many of our aches and pains.

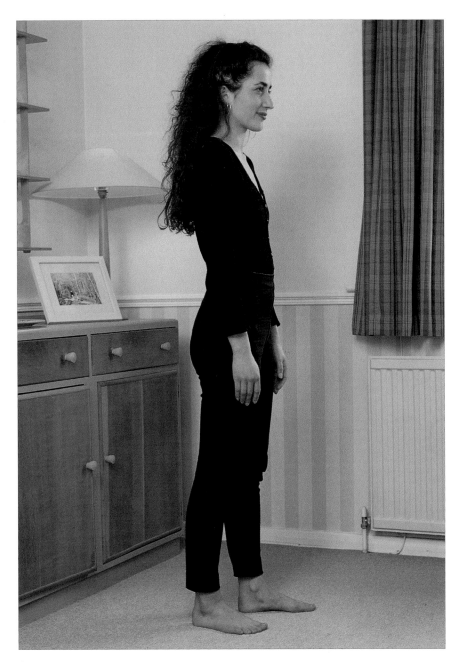

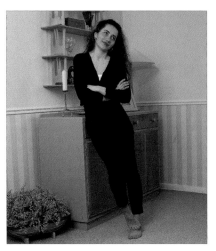

Below. *The automatic postural system supports and balances the body effortlessly, but because we unconsciously interfere with this system we often feel tired and need to prop ourselves up artificially by using objects around us. This woman not only has all her weight on one leg, but she is also leaning heavily on her right hip. This causes excessive wear and tear on the hip joint and may possibly result in the need for a hip operation in later life.*

Left. *If you are standing for any length of time it can be helpful to have your feet apart, one foot behind the other, at an angle of approximately forty-five degrees. This provides a more stable base, helping the body to maintain an upright posture with the minimum of effort. It will help you to think of your primary directions, and you could also think of releasing up in the front of the torso.*

Balance

When you are standing it is important to have the weight of your body on both feet, so make sure your knees are neither bent nor braced back. Many people adopt the habit of pulling their back in and pushing their pelvis forward, but this position is actually one of the most common causes of back pain while standing.

On the sole of each foot there are three points of contact with the ground:

- the heel
- the ball of the foot
- a point just below the little toe

These are the points that help us to achieve perfect balance. If we start to become aware that this is the case, we can direct our thoughts to our feet and allow them to spread more evenly on to the floor *(see overleaf)*. When the foot is spread more evenly on the ground, a stretch reflex reaction, which is situated in the sole of the foot, is stimulated. This reflex automatically affects the muscle fibres which in turn affect your posture by keeping you upright with the minimum amount of effort. So, simply by standing with equal weight on the three points of balance your posture will automatically improve.

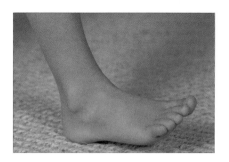

When you are walking, your heel should touch the ground first; this provides support for the next step. The weight should be slightly on the outside of the heel.

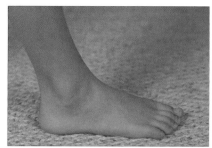

Then, as you move forward the whole foot rotates inwards so that it makes full contact with the floor. The three points of balance on the sole of the foot should now be bearing equal pressure.

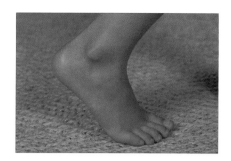

As you continue to move forward the reflexes in the foot cause your toes and the arch of your foot to act like a spring which carries you effortlessly into the next step.

Sitting

Many of the standard chairs we sit on slope backwards, inviting us to slump into them, and it makes it very difficult for us to maintain an upright posture without straining our bodies. When you think how much time we spend sitting down – in our cars, for our meals, at work or in front of the television, for example – many of us spend up to ten or eleven hours on chairs each day, which accounts for more than sixty per cent of our waking life. This is why it is so important that we do not place undue stress on our muscular system while we are sitting if we are to prevent the onset of aches and pains in later life. It is important to realize, however, that sitting in any posture for a short period of time is generally not going to produce any ill effects: habitual repetition of the same posture does the damage.

Even many people who study ergonomics fail to realize that it is the pelvis which needs to be supported rather than the lumbar spine. In fact, the lumbar curve is not a fixed feature of the spine, and often when a child or baby is sitting you will find that their lumbar curve has disappeared entirely, leaving a completely straight back *(see picture on page 34)*.

If you do not have a forward-tilting chair you can buy a wedge-shaped cushion to put on your ordinary chair. These are relatively inexpensive and will turn any chair into a forward-sloping one *(see page 141 for details)*. Once you have become accustomed to this

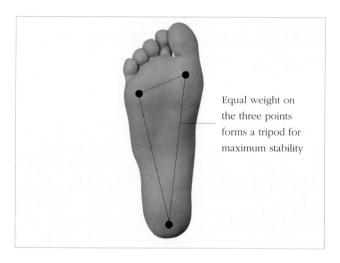

Equal weight on the three points forms a tripod for maximum stability

These three points form a tripod which maintains stability while standing, but it is common for people to put more weight on one or two of these points. This causes excessive tension as the muscular system overworks, trying to maintain balance.

new sitting position you will find that you can sit for longer periods with greater ease and increased comfort.

Driving

Car seats can cause back problems for the same reason. For example, bucket seats (particularly common in sports cars) encourage a very slumped posture, which exerts great pressure on the pelvic joints. It is ironic that the lumbar support in cars that feels so comfortable on a short trip is actually the cause of severe back problems on longer journeys. Many car seats have a lumbar curve built in, yet when sitting the lumbar spine naturally

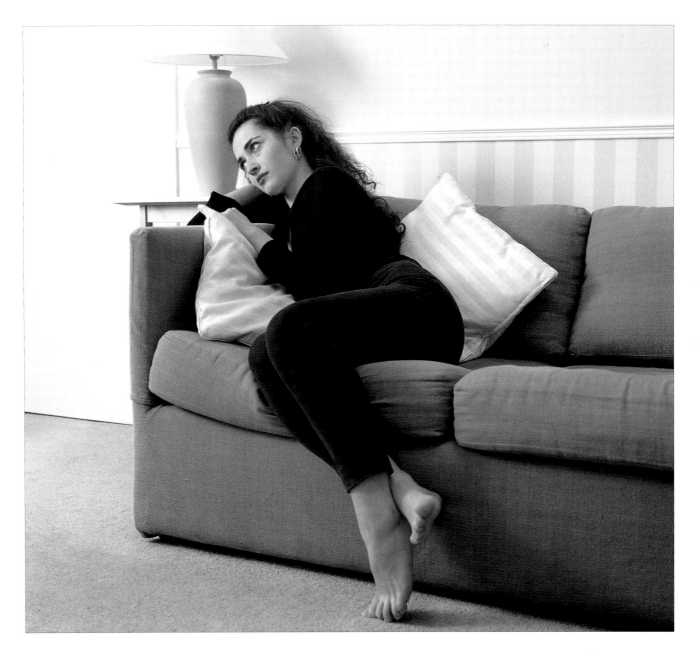

flattens; by artificially causing the lower spine to arch on long journeys it places it under enormous strain.

If you have enough headroom, then a wedged cushion may be suitable; if not, a triangular piece of foam placed in the area where the back of the seat meets the base will give your pelvis the support it needs which, in turn, will help the entire spine and head to be poised. At first, the new driving position may feel strange, but you will get used to the new posture within a week or so. You should also make sure that your seat is correctly adjusted, so that you do not have to strain in order to reach the steering wheel or the pedals.

This is a common way of sitting that can easily become a habit and can start to feel 'comfortable', yet the whole body is completely twisted out of alignment. Over long periods a strain is placed on most of the muscles, joints and internal organs, as well as the blood system itself – for example, the feeling of 'pins and needles' may arise where the flow of blood is constricted. Habitual repetition of this posture is likely to result in the inefficient working of most of the bodily systems.

Tension while driving is reflected in the way that people clench the wheel, erratically change gear and even grind their teeth. A little awareness can help to reduce the tension and ensure that it does not persist even when we have left the car *(see page 62).*

Walking

Often fashionable clothes and shoes can restrict movement and consequently affect co-ordination and balance. High-heeled shoes are among the worst offenders, and if worn for long periods of time over a number of months they can cause the muscles that run down the back of the leg to shorten. This can result in the inability of the person's heel to touch the ground when barefoot because the calf muscles are severely over-tightened. This affects the balance of the entire body as the three points of balance should be in contact with the ground to achieve maximum stability. When only two points make contact, stability is obtained by muscle tension instead of natural balance. Tight trousers, skirts or jeans can also affect the length of stride and even constrict our breathing. It is difficult to direct ourselves successfully if we have physical restrictions placed on us.

As in other activities, the way the body is designed to move is to lead with the head when walking. Just observe a young child and you will notice that when they see something they want, their eyes go towards the object of interest; since their eyes are in their head, and the weight of the head starts the movement, the rest of the body simply follows. Our thoughts affect the

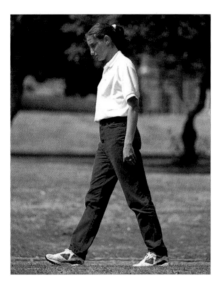

Above. *This woman's body has a downward direction because she is letting her head hang while she is deep in thought. As the head alone weighs approximately 6.5 kg (15 lb), this is likely to result in neck tension, and she may find that she also suffers from back problems, as her entire body has to work harder for any movement to occur.*

Right. *The same woman is now aware of what is going on around her and as a result her head is poised on top of her spine which encourages her body to be more erect. Simply by applying her primary directions, this change in awareness means that walking will be a less tiring experience for her.*

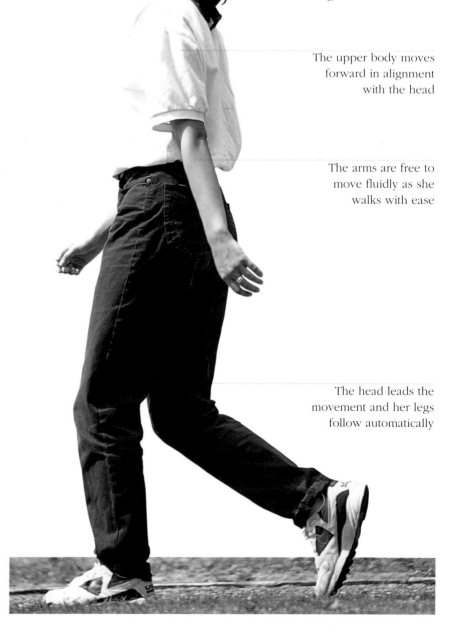

The upper body moves forward in alignment with the head

The arms are free to move fluidly as she walks with ease

The head leads the movement and her legs follow automatically

Right. *Notice how this woman is pulling herself down while walking upstairs. This downward pressure is counter to the direction of movement, and so results in the need for more muscular effort to achieve the task. The most noticeable tension will be in her leg muscles, as she has to push down into the ground to propel herself forward.*

Below. *By applying her directions – thinking of freedom in her neck muscles, letting her head go forward and up and allowing her spine to lengthen – she is able to walk up the steps with greater ease and efficiency. There is now much less strain on her leg muscles, and she will feel far lighter.*

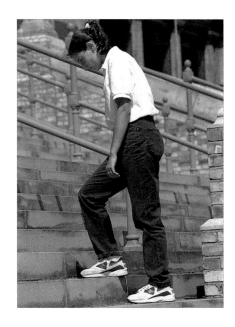

Below. *When walking down the steps this woman is letting her head hang downwards. Because the head is so heavy, the entire muscular system is overworked in an attempt to prevent her from falling forward down the steps. If this is done habitually, it could result in stiffness or even arthritis.*

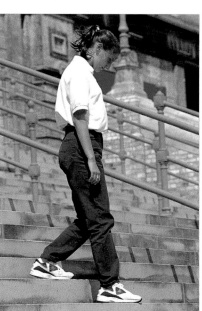

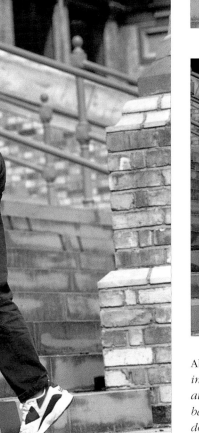

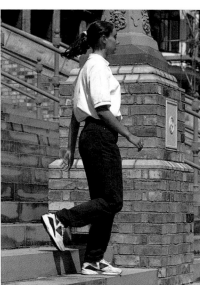

Above. *By thinking of lengthening up in front of her body and by being attentive of the head being finely balanced on top of the spine, walking downstairs automatically becomes easier. The entire movement becomes more poised and graceful; some people even describe this sensation as 'walking on air'.*

DRIVING

Right. *The backward-sloping seats in most modern cars encourage poor posture. Notice how this driver's lower back is sloping backwards yet his upper back is going forwards. As a result, he is bending his back in the middle, which puts his back under great strain; it should be the hip joints that rotate him forward towards the wheel. This is one of the reasons why large numbers of people tend to suffer from back pain and neck tension even after relatively short journeys.*

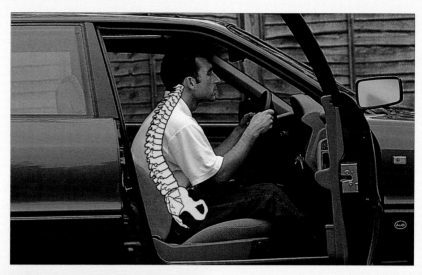

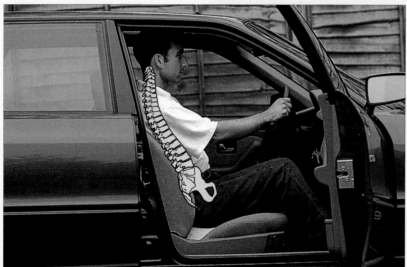

Left. *Simply by using a wedge-shaped cushion we can greatly improve our posture – the pelvis is now supported, which helps the spine to maintain its alignment. In this position the body is not under excessive strain and, in turn, this should make you feel more relaxed and able to cope with any stressful situations you may encounter on your journey. Make sure that your seat is fairly upright and that you leave plenty of time so you do not have to rush. Try not to grip the wheel too tightly, and you may also find it useful to be attentive to your breathing from time to time.*

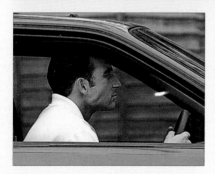

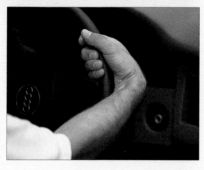

Whenever we are late for work or trying to meet important deadlines the 'fear reflex' is stimulated – the head retracts back on to the spine and the shoulders become arched. You can see how this driver is also gripping the wheel and clenching his jaw. If this happens often enough this tension remains with us even when we are not under stress.

Even placing your hands in awkward positions can produce unnecessary strain on fingers, wrists and shoulders. You can see that this driver's hand and forearm are almost at right angles: this places the wrist under an enormous amount of strain, which will give rise to tension in the arm muscle or even arthritis of the wrist if this position is adopted frequently.

COMMON CAUSES OF TENSION WHILE DRIVING

If you are aware of how tension can arise, you will be better prepared to deal with it:

- *We have to deal with a number of different stimuli at the same time.*
- *We have to react very quickly to these stimuli.*
- *Our 'fear reflex' is constantly triggered, as we are agitated time after time by other drivers on the road.*
- *We are often trying to get somewhere on time.*

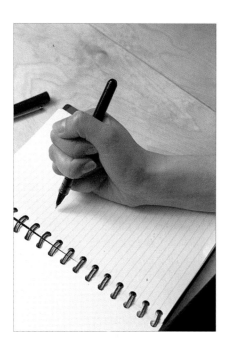 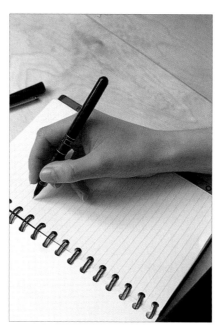

Far left. *You can see the tension in this woman's hand as she grips the pen very tightly. This tension can be present in the shoulder and neck, which may also be where it originates in the first place. This is often the cause of arm and shoulder problems, including writer's cramp, and could possibly also be the cause of repetitive strain injury.*

Left. *If you think of holding the pen gently with the minimum of tension, you will be less likely to suffer strain which can result in arthritis of the hands and fingers later on in life. You may also find that your handwriting improves; if you free your neck this will allow your shoulder, arm and wrist to move more fluidly, resulting in less tension in the hand and fingers.*

way we move – many of us walk around thinking about the past and the future and are very rarely engaged in what is happening in the present moment. In fact, most of us do not even look where we are going; we simply follow orders from our mind and do not give our senses and reflexes a chance to work.

Writing

It is amazing how some people hold their pens when writing! Both the position of the hand and the amount of muscle tension involved in the act of writing can cause muscular strain. Most problems usually stem from experiences at school, where children often have to write quickly in order to keep up in lessons. The direction of allowing the wrist, elbow and shoulder to be free and release away from each other can be particularly helpful here, and should help you to write with fluidity of movement as you guide the pen freely across the paper. Always remember to apply your primary directions first – this is necessary in order to be able to release tension in other areas of your body.

Working at a computer

It is easy to become so involved in your work that you give little or no attention to the strain you are putting yourself under while you perform a task. This can lead to your body being very tense for long periods, especially when there are important deadlines to meet. People often adopt a particularly bad posture when working at a computer, as they tend to hunch over the keyboard and peer forward to look at the screen. You need to think of releasing up in the front of your body from your navel up to your collar bone, and of not pulling your head back on to your spine *(see overleaf)*. When sitting for long periods it is important to have both feet on the ground because there are reflexes in the feet that affect your posture.

Reading

As many of us often read for fairly long periods of time without moving, it is especially important to sit in a position that does not put any of our muscles under excessive strain. You may sit curled up on the sofa, or hunch your shoulders in order to bring the book closer towards your head. You may also find that you lean your head to one side without realizing it – and then you wonder why you have a pain in your neck when you stop reading! It is vitally important that you are aware of how you are sitting if you are to avoid a number of common aches and pains. If you spend just a few moments being aware of your sitting posture before you start reading you are likely to have fewer problems after you finish.

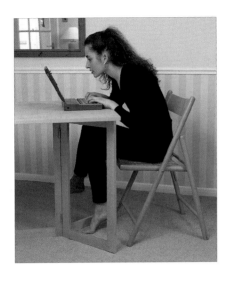

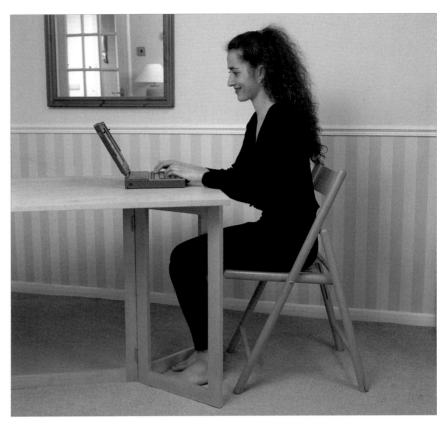

Above. *This woman is so involved with the information on the screen that she is totally unaware of her posture. Her legs are crossed which causes her pelvis to rotate. The toes of her right foot are supporting the weight of both legs, the top of her back is rounded and her head is rotating back, due to tension in the neck muscles.*

Above. *Being aware of how you are using your body can help to prevent a build-up of tension. This woman is resisting the urge to strain forward to look at the screen and her head is now poised on top of her spine. Also, both her feet are flat on the floor, allowing the reflexes in her feet to work to full effect.*

Inset. *This woman is sitting with her legs twisted one around the other, causing her whole body to be thrown out of alignment. This position is regarded by some as elegant, yet it may produce excessive tension in the legs, lower back and neck.*

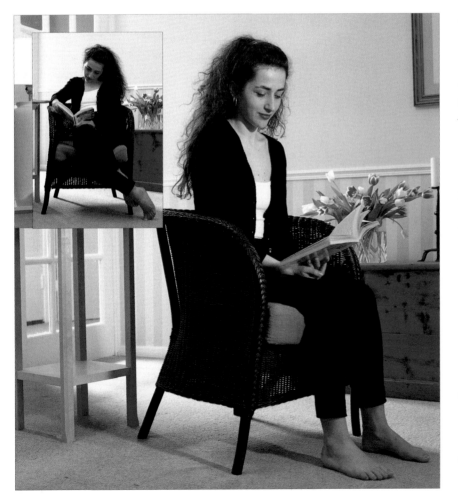

Left. *When sitting for long periods while reading, it is beneficial to have your head, spine and pelvis in alignment so that they support one another. If you position your legs so that your knees are directly above your feet, this also gives your legs support, and can help to alleviate stress in the lower back muscles.*

AN 'END-GAINING' ATTITUDE

Below. *Always being in a hurry has caused this woman to have an 'end-gaining' attitude. She is only concerned with getting the food and drink in her mouth before rushing off to her next appointment. She is not giving any thought to the way she is eating. Not only is her head being forcefully pulled back on to her spine, squashing the intervertebral discs, shortening her whole torso and compressing her stomach, but she is also unlikely to be enjoying her meal.*

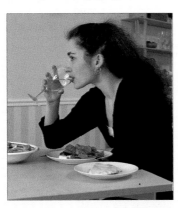

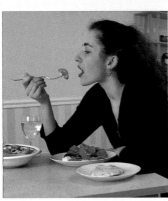

Right. *Just by allowing herself to slow down, her muscular system can become more relaxed. This naturally encourages better poise and balance and gives her the time to observe her movements so that she is aware of what she is doing.*

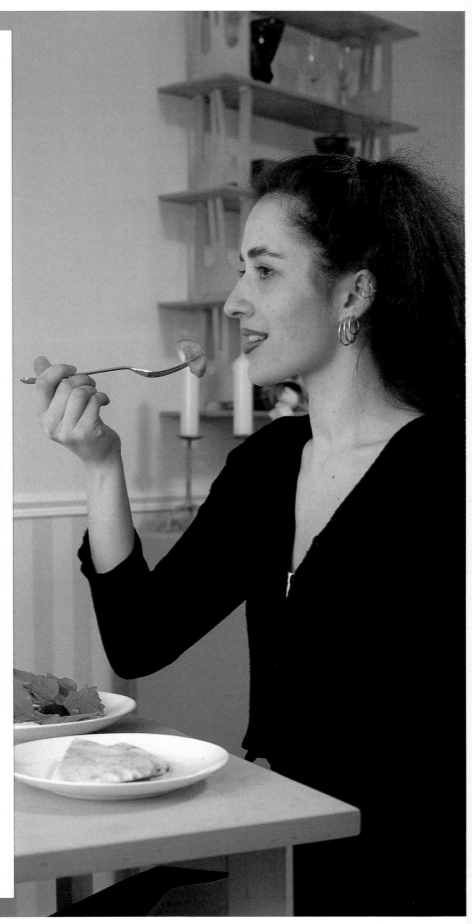

Generally, it is beneficial to change position about every ten to fifteen minutes, as even the best position may cause problems if held for long periods. It is important to realize that the Alexander Technique is not about 'dos' and 'don'ts', but is simply about being aware of what your body is doing at any given moment, and whether it is causing aches that can develop into more serious problems later on in life.

Eating and drinking

Even the way we eat and drink can affect the primary control of the body. Many of us are in a hurry when we eat, and are often only concerned with getting the food in our mouths as quickly as possible! We tend to move our head forward to meet the food, rather than bringing the food up to our mouth so that our head can remain poised above our spine. Even when eating and drinking we need to apply our primary directions and also keep both feet flat on the floor to allow our postural reflexes to work. It is especially important to maintain a good posture, as this can help the digestive system to function properly; eating in a hunched position can cause indigestion.

Playing musical instruments

The way musicians hold their instruments can cause many problems, such as neck and shoulder tension, backache and sciatica. It is not uncommon for professional musicians to have to give up their careers because of aches

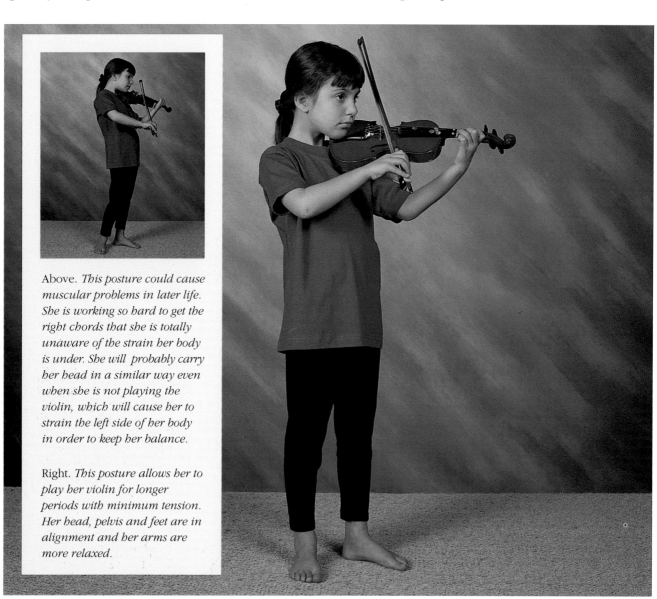

Above. *This posture could cause muscular problems in later life. She is working so hard to get the right chords that she is totally unaware of the strain her body is under. She will probably carry her head in a similar way even when she is not playing the violin, which will cause her to strain the left side of her body in order to keep her balance.*

Right. *This posture allows her to play her violin for longer periods with minimum tension. Her head, pelvis and feet are in alignment and her arms are more relaxed.*

Below. *Notice how this young musician is hanging her head down to meet the flute while throwing her pelvis to the left as the top half of her body is thrown to the right. Many hours of practising like this can not only produce severe muscle tension but can also affect her quality of playing.*

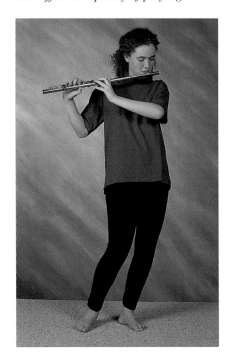

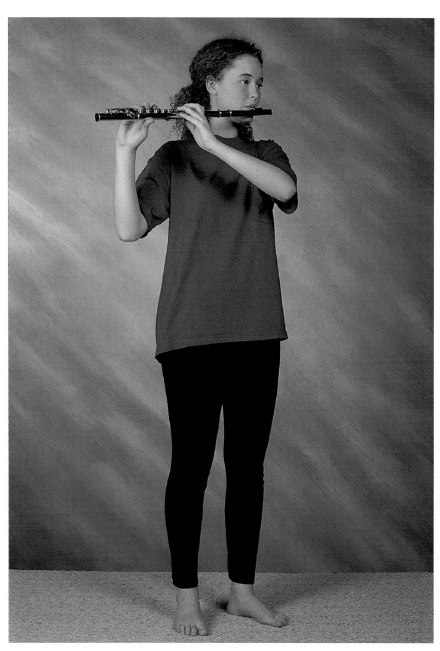

Right. *After some Alexander Technique lessons the girl is able to pay attention to the way she is standing and is able to apply her primary directions as well as thinking of her shoulders widening away from one another. This helps to release the tension that was caused by the awkward way that she held her flute previously.*

and pains caused by the way they stand or sit while playing, or by the way they grip their instrument. In our effort to achieve our goals we often lose the ability to succeed by trying too hard. From an early age children need to be taught how to use their bodies while playing their musical instrument so that they will not suffer later on in life. Once the primary directions have been applied, musicians can apply whichever secondary directions are most appropriate to their particular musical instrument, such as piano players allowing their hands to widen and their fingers to lengthen, for example.

A technique for every day

You can apply the principles of the Alexander Technique to every activity you perform, and although it may be difficult at first to be frequently aware of your movements, it becomes much easier as time goes on. Your body will soon become used to the new ways of moving. By being more conscious of the way your body moves, you also become more attentive and appreciative of everything in your environment and you will find that you have a greater enjoyment of life as your awareness of being in the present moment increases.

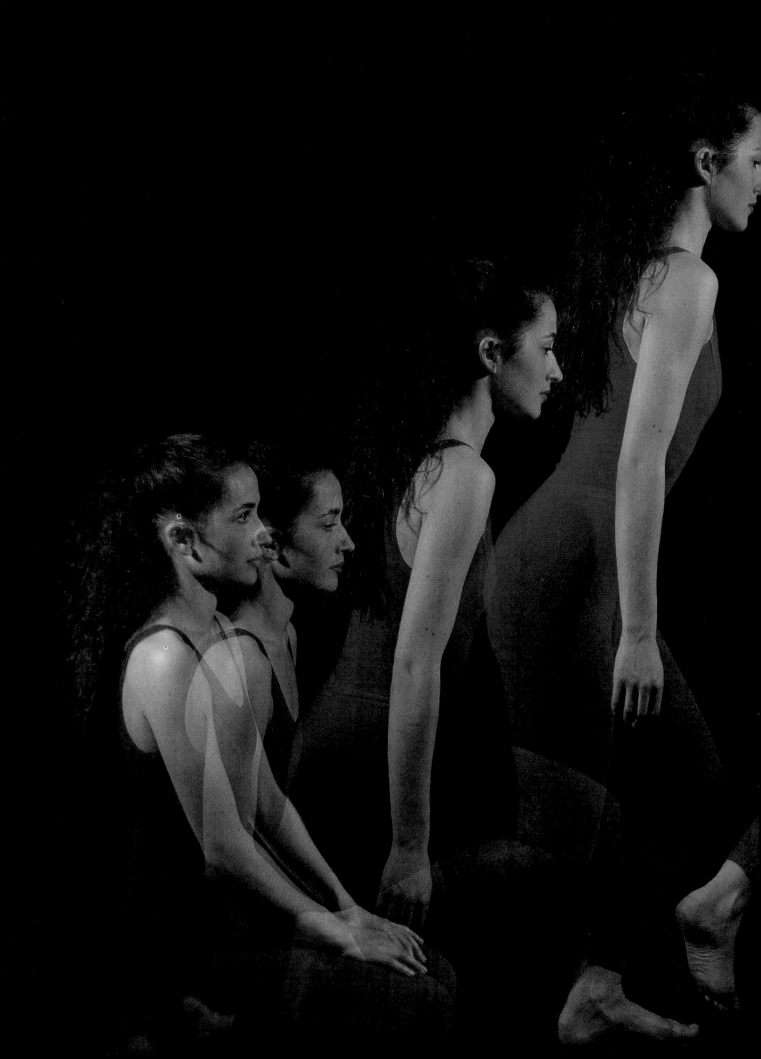

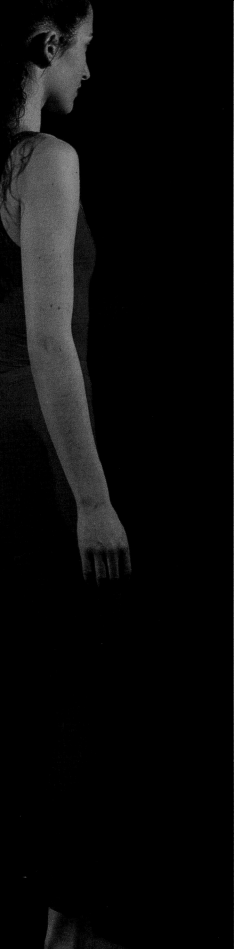

CHAPTER FIVE

First steps to reducing stress and tension

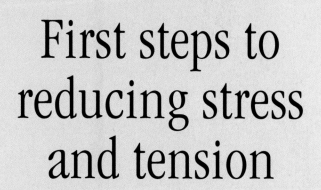

*'To be what we are, and to become
what we are capable of becoming, is the
only end of life.'*

Robert Louis Stevenson

*The best way to release unwanted muscular tension
is by lying on the floor. Getting up from the ground with
awareness can help your body to stay more aligned and
also help you to retain the benefits just achieved by lying
down. Being aware of the tension you hold in your
body is the first all-important step to reducing it.*

First steps to reducing stress and tension

As I have already mentioned, the pace of life in our society is becoming faster and faster and with it comes ever-increasing muscle tension as we try to cope with numerous stimuli every day. Even going back just fifty years, people were more relaxed and had more time for one another; television, and all the advertising that it brought with it, had not yet made a significant impact on people's lives. It is often very rare for us to be alone with our own thoughts, and we are encouraged from an early age to achieve more and more until many of us become 'human doers', rather than human beings.

The first step in letting go of unwanted tension is to stop completely and become aware of the tension you are holding within your muscles; it is not until you become aware of such tensions that you can do anything about them. Self-awareness is the fundamental tool that will help you to eradicate many of the ailments that life's stresses and strains have brought about.

Self-awareness exercise

Choose a quiet time of day when you can be alone. It does not matter whether it is early in the morning, during the day or in the evening. Spend ten minutes focusing on your body; you can start with your feet and work upwards. As you are being aware of your feet, try to release any tension that you can feel in your toes or ankles. Take as much time as you feel you need with any particular part of your body. At first, the ten minutes may feel like a long time, but as the days go by it will begin to seem shorter and shorter. You may find that your mind wanders off into other thoughts; if it does, do not get annoyed, just bring it gently back to the present moment by re-focusing your attention. Practise being the observer of your body, mind and emotions.

This exercise can be done either sitting or lying down, whichever feels more comfortable.

It is just as important to get in contact with how you are feeling and what you are thinking, as this will invariably affect levels of stress within your body. You could ask yourself the following questions:

1. *How am I feeling? Do I feel happy, sad, joyful, miserable, angry or any other emotion?* Perhaps you are feeling a lack of emotion. Try not to judge your feelings – there is no such thing as a bad emotion, although we may have had a negative reaction to an emotion that we have expressed in the past.

2. *Where do my thoughts wander off to? Do I have some concern or worry that is preoccupying my thoughts?* If you do, try to let your worries go just for these ten minutes.

When you have got used to this first exercise, you may like to try lying down in the 'semi-supine' position. This way of lying down has become the hallmark of the Alexander Technique. The word 'supine' simply means lying flat on the ground facing upwards. You will often find people who practise the Technique in this position!

The semi-supine position

The following procedure can be very effective in reducing the muscular tension that stress causes as well as increasing your vitality after a busy working day. It is particularly good for backache, neck problems and poor posture as it can help to align the spine and release tension in the neck and shoulders if it is done regularly. When getting into position, it is best to lie down by following the reverse of the sequence shown for getting up from the floor *(see page 76)*, as this puts your body under the least possible strain.

The purpose of this exercise is to release any excessive muscular tension throughout the body. It is one of the best positions for

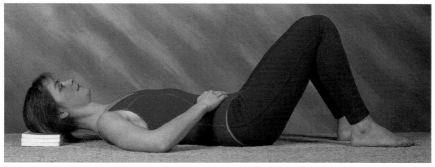

Left. *Lie down on your back and place some paperback books under your head. The books ensure that your head is supported, allowing your neck muscles to relax (your Alexander teacher will show you the exact height of books you need). They also encourage your head to go forward, causing a lengthening of the entire spine. Bend your knees so that they are pointing up to the ceiling; this allows your lower back to release (do not try to force your lower back to touch the floor – this will happen gradually). Bring your feet near to your pelvis, but make sure you are not straining your muscles by doing so. Both your feet should be making even contact with the floor so that all the reflexes are fully functional.*

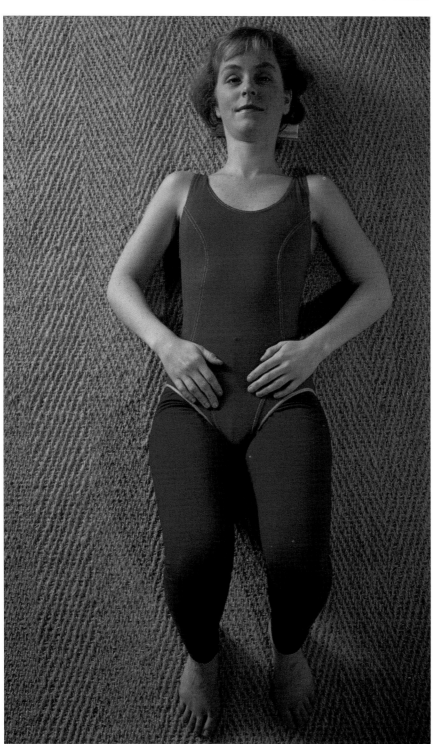

Left. *Place your hands gently on either side of your navel. It is good to have your hands in this position because it helps the shoulders to release away from one another. Make sure that there is some space between your feet, and enough space between your knees so that your legs do not fall inwards or outwards.*

71

releasing tension in the neck and shoulder area, as well as alleviating or preventing lower back pain. It is easier to let go of tension when lying down because gravity is working on your body in a different way and there is no chance of you falling over. The height of the books under the head will vary from person to person and, in some cases, from week to week. The best way to find the exact height is to ask your Alexander teacher when you start having lessons, but as a rough guide you can follow the instructions given above.

As Alexander discovered, most of us pull our heads back habitually without realizing it; the books underneath your head will, to some extent, stop this from happening. When first trying the semi-supine position you might like to place a thin piece of foam or a towel on top of the books so that they do not feel so hard; as the weeks progress you should find that you can discard it without any discomfort.

To begin with, you should follow the same procedure as for the previous exercise – just be aware of any tension you can feel. Compare the left side of your body with the right side to see if they feel symmetrical. This procedure

is known as 'active lying down', and although your body is in a state of rest it is not merely about resting; you are actively releasing tension by giving directions. You should be in a heightened state of awareness with your eyes open, so make sure that you do not fall asleep!

As you learn how to release tension, your lower back will gradually flatten on to the ground; this might take weeks or even months to happen, so please be patient with yourself. Many of these tensions have taken years to accumulate – they are not going to disappear overnight. Always make sure that the soles of your feet are in contact with the floor. There are powerful reflexes in the feet which activate postural muscles throughout the body, and even though you are resting these can still be in operation. If the postural muscle fibres are activated, the activity muscles can then release more easily.

Applying your directions

Here are just a few directions that will help you to release unwanted muscular tension whilst lying in the semi-supine position. It is important to remember that you must not 'do' anything to find the right position – the process of releasing tension actually depends

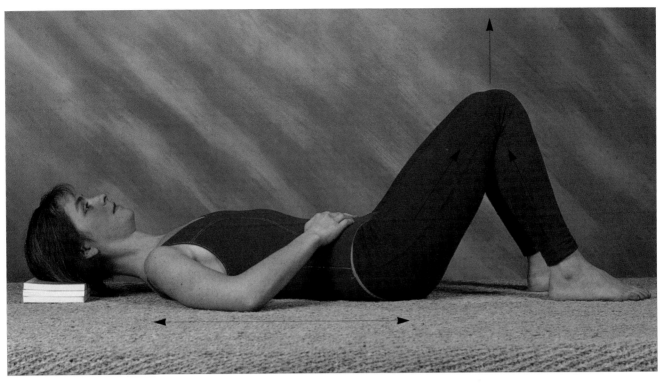

● Think of your head going forward and outward away from your spine. *This helps to release neck tension and also helps the spine to lengthen. You may not 'feel' anything happening but your muscles will be releasing without your conscious knowledge.*

● Think of your entire back lengthening and widening on to the floor. *It is very important that you do not 'do' anything to make this happen as this will only tighten up the back muscles, which is the opposite of what you are trying to achieve.*

● *Release the tension in your legs by imagining your knees going up to the ceiling. You may like to think of your knees being held up by imaginary strings attached to the ceiling. Remember to use only your thoughts, rather than muscular tension, to achieve your goal.*

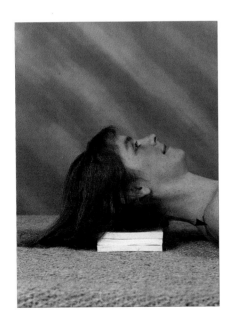

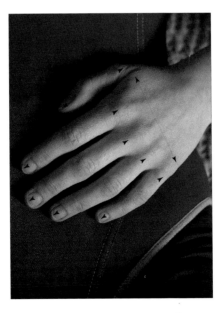

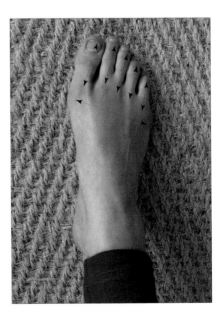

● Allow your neck muscles to lengthen *so that any excess tension in the neck is released. This will free your head from your spine, which is essential if you are going to apply directions successfully to other areas of your body.*

● *Let go of any tension in your fingers, hands and wrists by* allowing your fingers to lengthen and the palms of your hands to widen. *Make sure you only think of these directions and do not use your hand or finger muscles.*

● Allow your toes to lengthen as the soles of your feet spread out on to the floor. *This will help you to let go of any tension in your toes and feet. This is a common place of tension that many people are completely unaware of.*

● Think of your elbows releasing away from one another. *This will help to free the wrist and elbow joints as well as helping to release tension in and around the shoulders. Make sure there is sufficient space between your elbows and rib-cage, otherwise there will be excess tension in the wrists and the shoulders will start to hunch and become rounded.*

● Think of your left shoulder releasing away from your right hip and think of your right shoulder releasing away from your left hip. *These two directions can be very beneficial for releasing tension around the rib-cage and in the abdomen. The directions open out the front of the chest, which helps you to adopt a more upright posture.*

● Think of your shoulders widening away from one another. *This will release muscular tension in the upper part of the chest which will improve your breathing. This direction is particularly helpful to anyone with rounded shoulders and those who suffer from asthma.*

● Think of lengthening up the front of your body from your navel to the top of your chest. *Most of us have shortened muscles in the front of our body due to leaning over a desk at work or at school. This direction helps us to achieve a more upright posture with minimum effort.*

on you 'doing less'. It may take a few weeks or more before you feel totally comfortable with this new position, so do not worry if it feels a little odd at first.

Lie down in the semi-supine position as described above initially for ten minutes each day, and lengthen the time progressively by adding one minute a day until you have reached twenty minutes. If at any time you experience pain in your back or neck while lying down, stop immediately. Never push yourself; it is not an endurance test.

Your eyes should remain open throughout the exercise, and once you are used to the position you can start to think consciously of your muscles releasing tension. It is now time

for you to apply your directions *(see also chapter four)*, and the superimposed arrows on the previous page and this page show how the tension in your body releases. The directions are highlighted in the captions for maximum clarity.

Things to avoid

There are a number of common mistakes that people make when they first begin to do this exercise; these make it more difficult to release tension, and some even create new tension in the body (which is the opposite of what you are trying to achieve!). It is helpful to be aware of them when you are lying down, so you can make sure that you are lying in the correct position *(see opposite)*.

74

THINGS TO AVOID IN THE SEMI-SUPINE POSITION

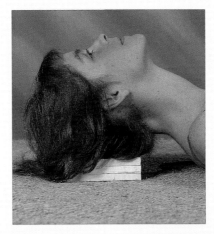
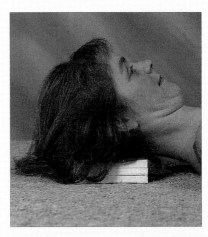

Right. *If you tend to pull your head back on to the books you might find it helpful to release the tension in the back of your neck by thinking of your chin dropping towards your chest.*

Far right. *It is easy to tuck in your chin rather than just to think of it dropping. This can increase neck tension and may even restrict breathing.*

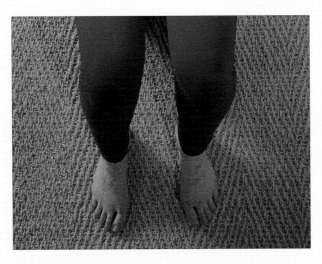

Above. *If you find that your legs tend to fall in towards each other or out away from each other, follow one of these instructions: if your legs tend to fall inwards, move your feet closer together; if your legs tend to fall outwards, move your feet further apart. You should end up with your feet more in line with your knees (as shown here). In this way your feet will support the weight of your legs, and you will be able to release muscle tension in your legs and lower back more effectively.*

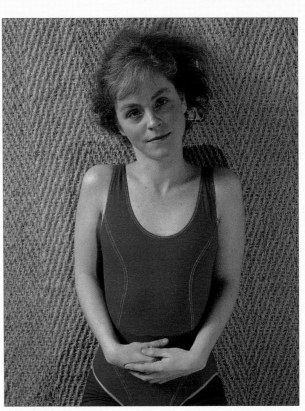

Above. *If you tuck your elbows into your ribs it makes it more difficult to release tension in your shoulders, elbows and wrists. Allow some space between your elbows and your rib-cage; you may like to think of your arms and ribs making an equilateral triangle.*

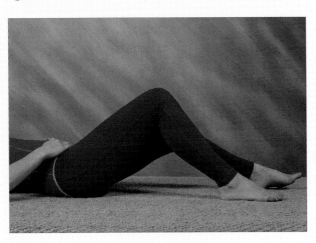

Left. *Your feet should be close to your pelvis without straining. If they are too far away (as shown here) it makes it harder to find a balanced position, and the lower back will not release so easily. It is also easy to go to the opposite extreme and pull your feet close in towards your buttocks. This puts unnecessary strain on the ankle, knee and pelvic joints, so defeating the whole purpose of the exercise.*

Getting up from the floor

It is important to be aware of the way you get up from the floor since you do not want to over-strain your muscles once you have released them. The following sequence is one of the easiest ways of standing up, which places the minimum strain on the body.

At first you may find that this way of getting up feels strange, but this is only because it probably goes against your habitual way of moving. Initially, it is important to perform the actions slowly to give yourself enough time to be aware of any tension within your body and to apply your directions. It can also be helpful to pause at any stage so that you have a chance to think about the next movement rather than just rushing into it. The sequence will become easier with practice, and soon you will find that it is almost second nature.

1 *Before you move, pause for a moment, and consciously decide on which side you are going to get up. Then look in that direction, but make sure you do not lift your head off the books in the process.*

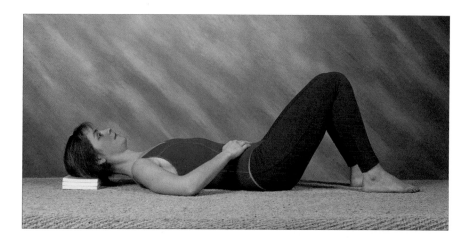

2 *Allow your head to roll on the books, following the direction of your eyes, and bring your arm over as shown. Then let your legs gently fall so that your entire body is moving in one direction.*

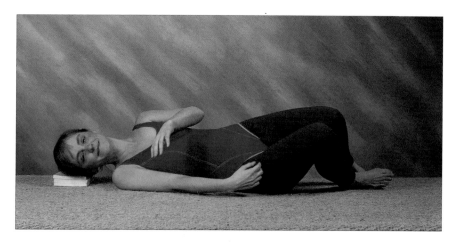

3 *You will be rolling on to one arm, but use the free arm to come over your body and support you as you lift your head from the books. This will avoid over-tensing your neck muscles.*

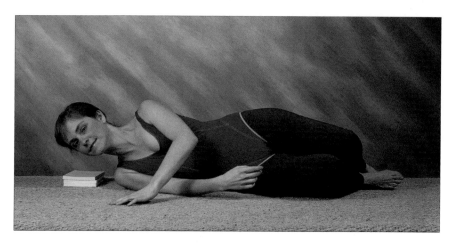

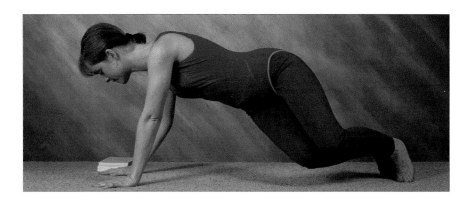

4 *Now support yourself with both hands keeping your arms straight, and press down with your toes. This will lift your knees from the ground so that you can bring them underneath your pelvis, enabling you to come on to all fours.*

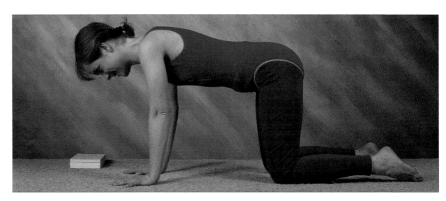

5 *Pause for a moment as this is a good resting position; be aware of your breathing and any excessive muscular tension that may have arisen during the last few movements. Simply pausing and being aware of tension will help to release it and will encourage your breathing to become deeper.*

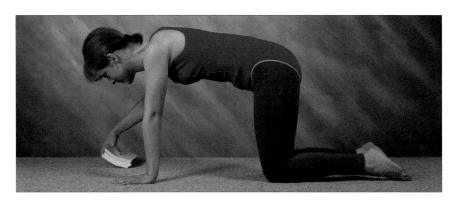

6 *It is common sense to pick up your books at this point as this will save you having to bend over for them once you are standing up, and perhaps tensing your muscles again in the process. It is easier to collect the books with the hand that is nearer to them.*

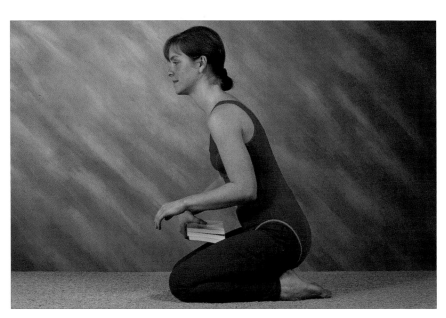

7 *Come back into a kneeling position so that for a moment you are sitting on your heels. Try to be aware of any tension in your neck and back, as this is another good resting place where you can pause and release any tension that you may feel.*

8 *While thinking of your head going forward and up, lean forward so that you come into a full kneeling position. In this posture your upper leg should form a ninety-degree angle with your lower leg. Now bring one foot forward in preparation for moving into the standing position.*

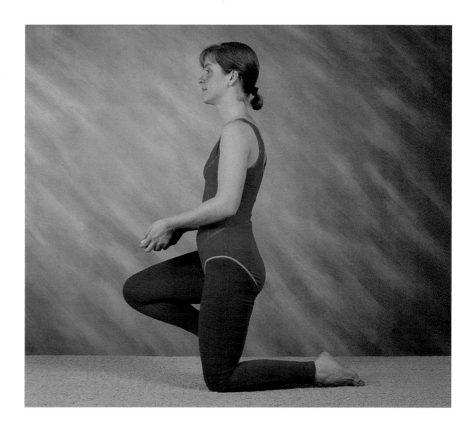

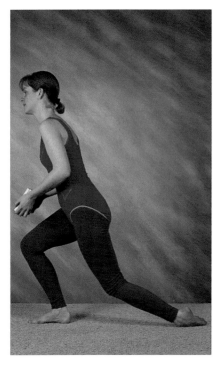

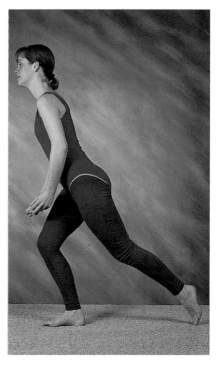

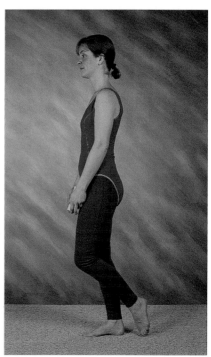

9 *Again, using the primary directions of allowing freedom in your neck, thinking of your head going forward and upwards and letting your spine lengthen, lean forward from your pelvis on to the foremost foot and this will naturally bring you into standing. You do not have to press your feet*

down hard on to the floor for this to happen – the postural reflexes in the feet are automatically activated when you lean forward. This will keep you in perfect balance naturally without any effort on your part. In this position, the weight of the head is balanced out by the weight of the left leg.

10 *This will bring you back into standing with the minimum amount of effort and you will be able to maintain the body's natural alignment that you achieved while lying down. Try to keep thinking of your directions as you go about your everyday activities.*

Benefits from lying in the semi-supine

Benefits will arise only if this exercise is done on a regular basis (if possible, once a day for at least ten minutes) over a period of some weeks. The best time to lie down is half-way through your day; if this is not always practical, try to lie down when you get home from work. Some people find that they sleep better if they lie in the semi-supine just before going to bed; others feel that starting the day in this way is more beneficial, as they can feel the effects throughout the whole day. It is better not to lie down after a heavy meal, as this will probably feel quite uncomfortable. Make sure you are warm enough, because it is much harder to release tension if you are feeling cold or lying in a draught. If necessary, place a blanket over yourself while you are lying down.

When you are lying down the spine is at rest; this is the best position in which to release any tension that has built up. When you are upright, the curves in the spine can sometimes be exaggerated, which can shorten your stature and have short- and long-term effects on the rest of your body. Being upright is not the problem in itself; it is the way in which we hold ourselves that puts the spine under so much pressure. Lying down in the semi-supine position once a day alleviates this pressure and prevents any tension from building up and causing harmful repercussions later on in life. In the short term, tiredness and fatigue can lead to the feeling that life is an effort and can make us feel irritable and depressed. In the long term, the spine can become deformed, as in the case of scoliosis (lateral curvature of the spine), spondylitis (arthritis of the spine) and Dowager's hump (excessive curvature around the seventh cervical vertebra – found mainly in elderly people, caused by stooping). Lying down for periods in the semi-supine position can help slow down the process of deterioration of the bones and joints of the spine, and even start to rejuvenate parts of the skeleton that have suffered from excessive wear and tear. You may also feel that you have more energy in the evening to do the activities that interest you.

MAIN BENEFITS FROM LYING IN THE SEMI-SUPINE POSITION

- *Release of muscular tension throughout your entire body.*
- *Lengthening of your spine so that it can support you better when you are upright.*
- *Improvement in your breathing as you are able to release tension around the rib-cage.*
- *Improved circulation (the blood can flow better through muscles that are relaxed). This also places less strain on the heart.*
- *Freer joints so that you are able to move with greater ease.*
- *Nerves that have become trapped due to over-tense muscles are freed.*
- *The internal organs have more room to function.*
- *A reduction in overall stress and tension physically, mentally and emotionally.*

Long-term effects

You may notice that your parents' or grandparents' height diminishes as they grow older. Many of us think that this is part of the normal ageing process, yet findings from experiments performed in the 1930s by a scientist called DePuky, a physician from Budapest, indicate otherwise. He discovered that the loss in height was due to the gradual loss of the fluid of which the intervertebral discs are largely made up. Therefore, this slight loss in height that many of us experience as we get older may partly be due to the undue pressure we exert on these discs while performing our daily activities throughout our lives (*see illustration on page 54*). Practising the semi-supine exercise each day helps to prevent any further deterioration of the discs, as it allows the spine to lengthen. If you do this exercise regularly over a few months you may even find that your height increases by 2–3 cm (1 in) or more.

Regular practice will help your muscles to remain relaxed for longer and longer periods, and you will find that you are more likely to remain calm when under pressure. You may also be less likely to suffer from arthritis caused by poor posture later on in life.

Remember: At first you may not feel the changes that are happening, so be patient and do not try to force your body to do anything.

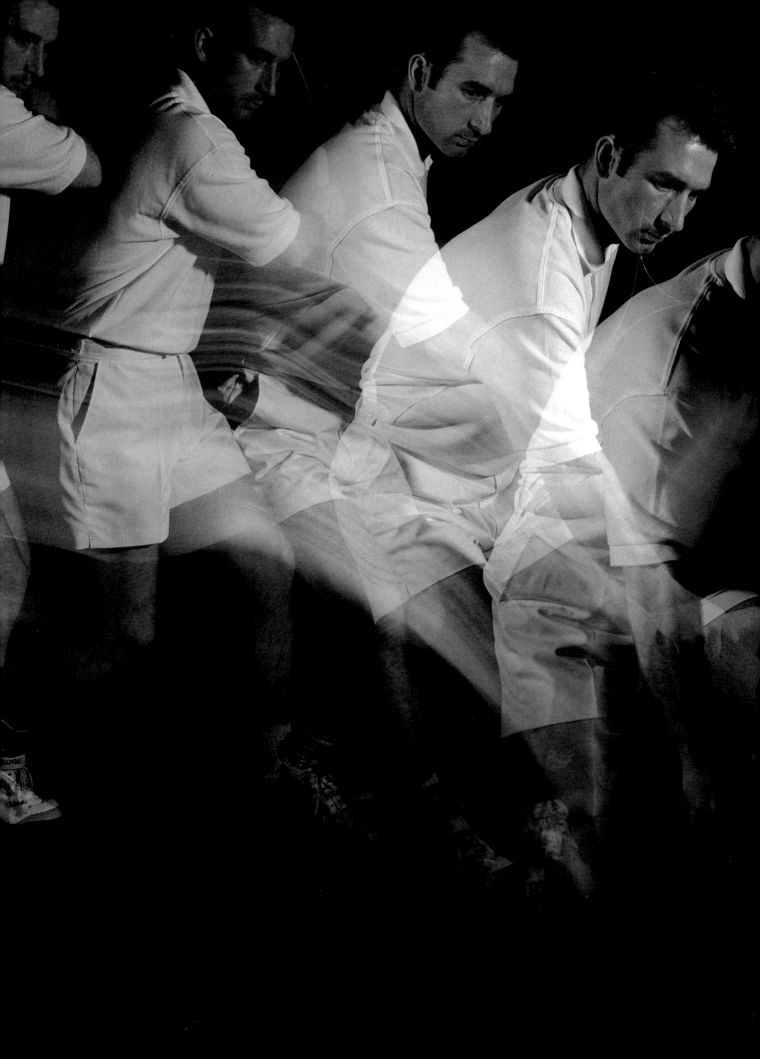

CHAPTER SIX

The Alexander Technique and sport

*'Knowing others is intelligence;
knowing yourself is true wisdom.
Mastering others is strength;
mastering yourself is true power.'*

Lao-tzu

*When playing any sport, if you apply the
principles of inhibition and direction you will feel
more relaxed and find the game more enjoyable. You may
even improve the quality of your game. This tennis player
moves fluidly as he reaches to hit the ball because he
is allowing his head to lead the movement.*

The Alexander Technique and sport

The Alexander Technique has helped all kinds of sportsmen and sportswomen, both at amateur level and in training for high-pressure competition. Since the way you use your body can affect the efficiency of your performance, it follows that the more aware you are of your actions, the greater the control you will have of your body. The Alexander Technique can be used effectively in a wide variety of different sporting activities, including horse riding, where the rider's posture clearly affects the performance of the horse, and in giving runners a new style of running that is not only more efficient, but also less strenuous.

Sport places greater demands on your body than normal everyday activities and can lead to injury in the form of twisted ankles, torn ligaments and sometimes even broken bones; using less tension in demanding activities can dramatically reduce the risk of injury to yourself. The increased freedom and flexibility that the Technique imparts can not only help to bring about improvements in performance, but also helps many people to experience renewed pleasure in their sport.

Most of the early training in various sports invites us to constantly try harder and harder, which can result in excessive muscle tension. This puts us under an enormous pressure which, if allowed to persist, can interfere with our natural mechanisms. This, in turn, can sometimes result in us giving up our favourite sport altogether. It is often hard, at first, for many of us to give up our old habitual way of straining, but when we do we are amazed to find that an easier, more flowing style can produce the same, or even better, results with less effort.

The importance of inhibition

People from unindustrialized societies seem to have the ability to perform enduring tasks with ease because they are not 'end-gaining' during their activities in the same way that we do in Western society. In her book, *The Continuum Concept*, psychotherapist Jean Liedloff, who lived with Stone Age Indians from South America, describes her insights into the way they go about their everyday actions. She noted that there was no sense of competition and they did not judge each other's performance of various tasks. Consequently, they were able to carry out their activities with greater ease and efficiency. They economized their energy by using the minimum required to accomplish the job, wasting none on associated tensions. This is exactly what the Alexander Technique sets out to achieve, and this principle is particularly important when it comes to sporting activities, where conservation of energy is of fundamental importance.

To many people involved in sport, the idea of not being goal-orientated is difficult to grasp because it goes against everything they have been taught in almost every aspect of their lives. To have the wish to achieve your end, yet at the same time to remain detached from it, is the secret of success and happiness and this is one of the core principles behind the Alexander Technique.

This 'standing back', or pausing before action, can also be seen in aikido, judo, tai chi and other martial arts that have been practised in the East for thousands of years. The true masters of their arts perform all actions with grace and beauty, yet at the same time with great power. The secret is to remain composed at all times and to give yourself time to perform the activity with ease. This principle is just as applicable in the middle of a football match, on the tennis court, on the ski slopes or in any of our Western sports.

Active awareness

Another major problem stems from our faulty sensory perception which gives us false information about where our body is in space. This can obviously have a significant effect on any sporting activity: if you think you are in one position when you are actually in another, then your co-ordination and balance will obviously be affected. This can be the reason why even the greatest athletes sometimes make silly mistakes, especially under pressure when there is bound to be more tension in their muscles, generating stress throughout the body. In fact, it is common to see both amateur and professional sportspeople with teeth clenched, lips pursed and forehead frowning in the effort to win; however, as a consequence of over-tightened muscles, movements become awkward, therefore diminishing the chances of performing well.

By applying the principles of the Alexander Technique we can start to correct our old habitual movements that produce these tensions, and replace them with more poised and fluid ways of moving. By becoming more aware of both ourselves and our surroundings we can gain a greater conscious control over our bodies, thus increasing our chances of performing well.

The road to success

As any sportsperson will tell you, there is also a very important psychological aspect, which can make the difference between winning or losing a game or race; even the best players might play well one day and badly the next for no obvious reason. The calmer and more detached you are, the greater your chances of success will be. By practising inhibition and direction you will find that your mind is in a better state to cope with the pressure of the game, at whatever level you are playing. It will also help you to remain calm once you have made a mistake, rather than allowing it to escalate into a series of disasters that can often cost you the game.

It is frequently the case that the harder you try the worse things get. The secret is to let your body move with the natural ease and agility that lies beneath your postural habits and conditioned ways of performing activities. Most important of all is to enjoy the sensation

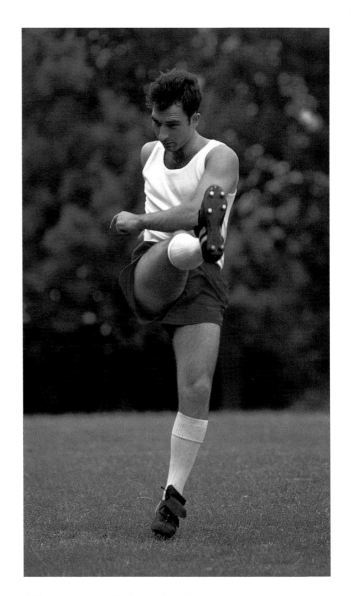

When your mind is focused in the present moment your body is more at ease and your chances of success are greatly improved as a result. You will also get more pleasure out of your game, whether you win or lose.

of every action, because when you are happy with your body's performance you will attain an excellence that is not only rewarding for you, but is also a pleasure to watch. If you observe the great athletes, whether their sport is ice-skating, running, snooker or football, you will see that they perform their actions with incredible ease; comments like 'they make it look so easy' can often be heard whenever they perform.

The following pages feature a variety of sports and show you some of the ways in which the Alexander Technique can help you to improve your performance.

Golf

A common sight on the golf course is a rounded spine and knees that are braced backwards. Many golfers are completely unaware that the way they stand while hitting the ball can affect the quality of their game. A common fault in golf is the inability of the player to keep their eye on the ball – this is absolutely vital to achieving an accurate shot. It is very easy to become distracted at the crucial moment and to let your mind wander (Alexander himself described this as the 'mind-wandering habit').

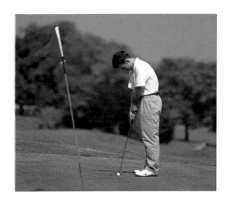

Above. *This golfer is much too near to the ball, which is why his style is very cramped. His back is curved and his knees are braced back, straining his entire body unnecessarily. This is because he has rushed into the shot without thinking.*

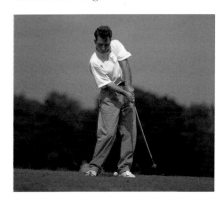

Above. *A front view reveals how out of balance the golfer is. His torso and head are going in the opposite direction to his legs, causing his muscular system to over-tense, which interferes with the natural flow of movement.*

Right. *When the teacher helps him to release tension in his neck muscles, his balance and co-ordination improve. His spine is straighter and his knees are bent, and he will be more able to succeed.*

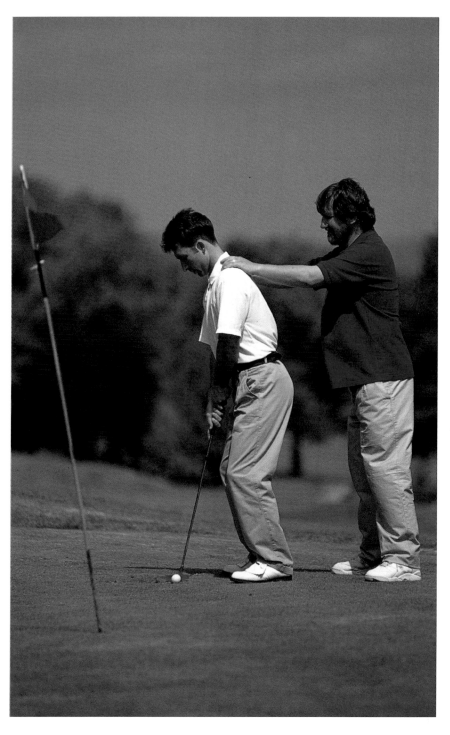

Below. *After some lessons the golfer is able to maintain the improved co-ordination by himself. He is no longer hunched over the ball and his head is poised on top of his spine, giving him the freedom to let his body move with ease. At first he will probably find this new stance very strange, but in time it will become much more comfortable than his old habit.*

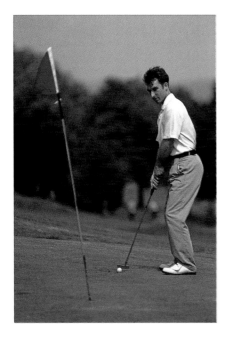

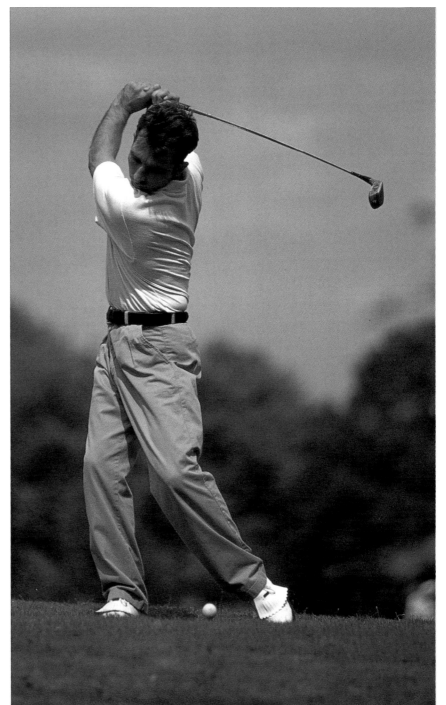

Right. *Notice the difference in the golfer's swing – there is now much more energy being directed into his drive. His whole body is hitting the ball rather than various parts of this body going in different directions. His torso and head are now above his legs so that his whole body is in balance and is more aligned. His muscles now do not have to tense in order for him to keep his balance.*

By practising inhibition and applying your primary directions you will be able to overcome many of the habits that are actually holding you back from becoming a better golfer. You will also be able to release and prevent excess tension in the body which could otherwise perhaps result in injury. For example, a common problem is golfer's elbow: this is caused by over-straining the wrist by either bending or twisting it continually, and results in pain on the inner side of the elbow. If you are aware of what you are doing, you will be able to give yourself directions to allow the freedom of movement that will help you to move with fluidity and ease. It is particularly important to have muscular freedom in your arms and shoulders, and by attending Alexander lessons you will find that your shoulders feel much looser, as though they are 'well oiled'.

Football

Football is a sport where injury is very common, particularly leg injury. You need to be aware not only of where you are in relation to the ball, but also of where the other players are, especially when they are about to tackle. For this, as in every other sport, inhibition is crucial. When you kick the ball awkwardly it is likely to cause tension within your body as well as perhaps resulting in an inaccurate kick. Only by pausing can you give yourself the time you need to take in all the information necessary to make a successful kick, whether it is to score a goal or to pass to another player.

Through the Alexander Technique you will be able to achieve a muscular system that is free, and which enables you to run, kick and jump with greater ease. This increased agility can be vital when it comes to outplaying your opponents in a tough match.

Right and below. *This footballer's lack of co-ordination severely affects his play – he is only concentrating on the ball and has completely forgotten to pay attention to his own movements. One minute he is on top of the ball because he has rushed in without having any spatial awareness – this gives him very little room in which to manoeuvre – and the next he is leaning away from the ball, causing all his muscles to overwork just to keep him from falling. As a consequence he is often out of balance, which causes him to kick the ball inaccurately. This, in turn, will make him annoyed with himself for missing an easy shot, which results in excessive muscular tension which will affect his play.*

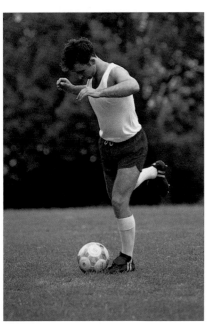

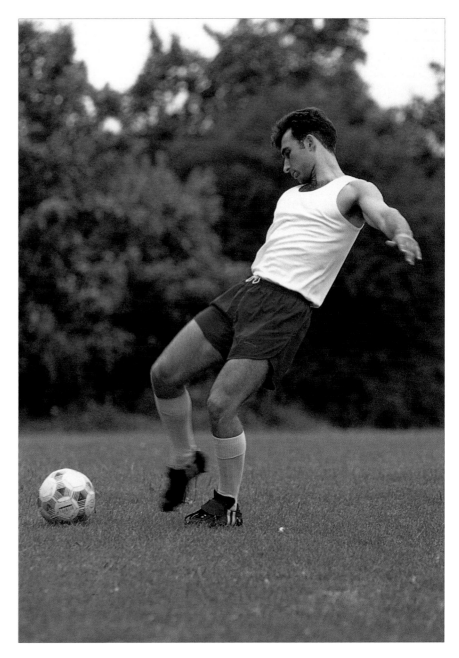

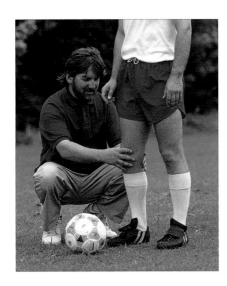

Above. *The Technique can help to release the tension in the knees, hips and ankle joints so that running and kicking put the body under less strain. The footballer will then be able to move more, freely which will greatly improve his style of play.*

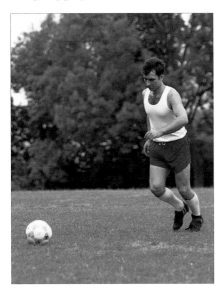

Above and right. *By having a series of Alexander lessons the footballer will learn practically how the head leads all movement. By applying the simple principles of inhibition and direction he will find that he is much less tired at the end of a game and he is kicking the ball with much more power and accuracy. In short, he will gain more control over both himself and the ball as he will be more aware of his movements.*

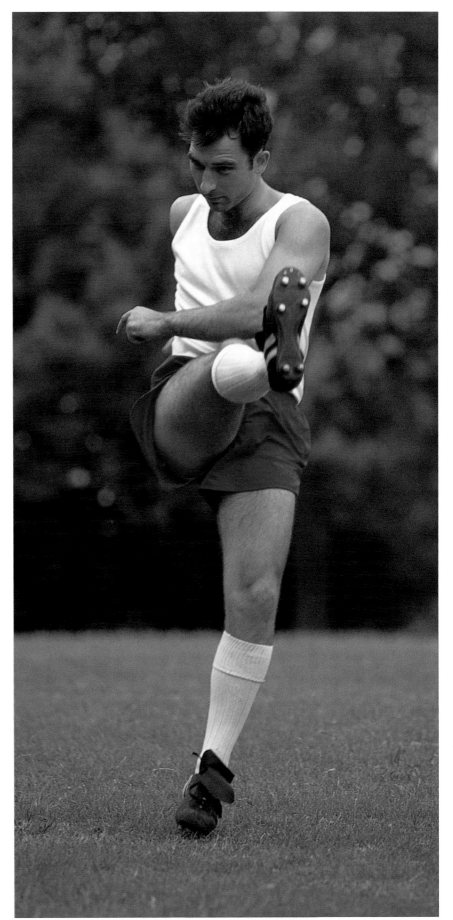

Horse riding

The Alexander Technique is often used by horse riders because their posture affects the horse's performance. The horse immediately responds to the movements the rider makes, and the more poised the rider is, the more graceful and efficient the horse's performance will be. I have taught several riders who complained that they found it difficult to get their horse to do as they wished – they usually blame the horse without even considering that their own posture may be interfering with the horse's movement. One of my students complained that her horse never went in a straight line, but after a few lessons she realized that she had actually been sitting off-centre, causing her horse to move to the right. When she was able to correct her posture, the horse did what she had wanted it to do all along!

By having Alexander lessons you will be more confident, and this confidence will naturally be transmitted to your horse, who will now instinctively know who is 'in charge'. This is vitally important when it comes to controlling your horse. Also, if you ever fall off your horse you will be less likely to hurt yourself if your muscles are relaxed, rather than in a state of tension due to fear or anxiety.

Right and below. This rider is leaning too far forward and gripping the reins too tightly because she is afraid of falling off. Her back is rounded as a result, and this throws her entire body out of alignment so that her weight is not distributed evenly in the saddle. It is interesting to see that when the rider drops her head and leans forward the horse also drops its head, and this will affect the way the horse performs.

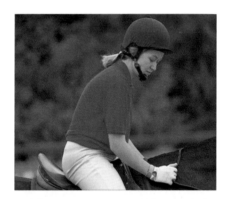

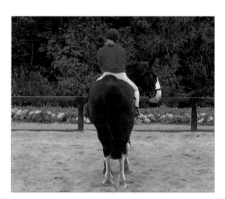

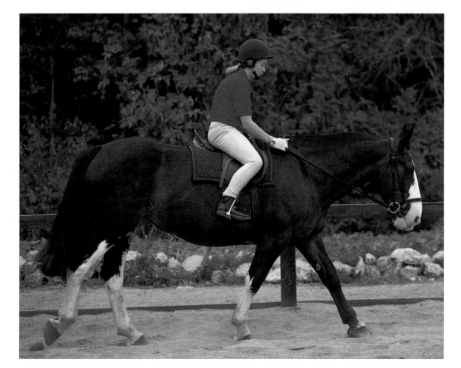

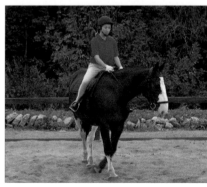

Top and above. If the rider is leaning to one side the horse will be inclined to go in the same direction. Because most of us suffer from a faulty sensory perception of ourselves, this rider thinks she is straight when she is not. Her unbalanced posture means that she will be more likely to fall off if the horse makes any sudden movements.

Right. *The Alexander Technique teacher minutely alters the rider's posture by bringing her head over the top of her spine and helping her back to lengthen, which releases muscular tension and brings her into alignment. Her faulty perception of herself is addressed so that she becomes more aware of the way she is sitting on the horse.*

Below and inset. *After Alexander lessons the rider sits much straighter with a lengthened back and her head poised on top of her spine. Her head, pelvis and heels are now aligned – this posture will help her to achieve the best response from her horse. Horse and rider now move as one entity in a more flowing style. Note that, because the rider's head is going forward and up, the horse's head has also lifted in response.*

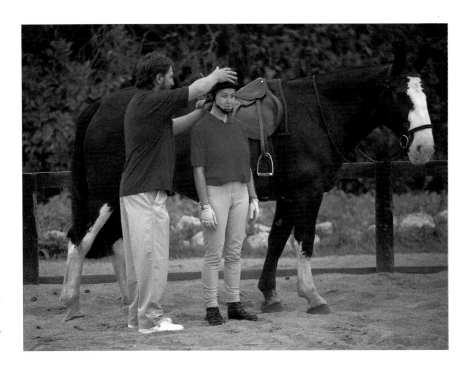

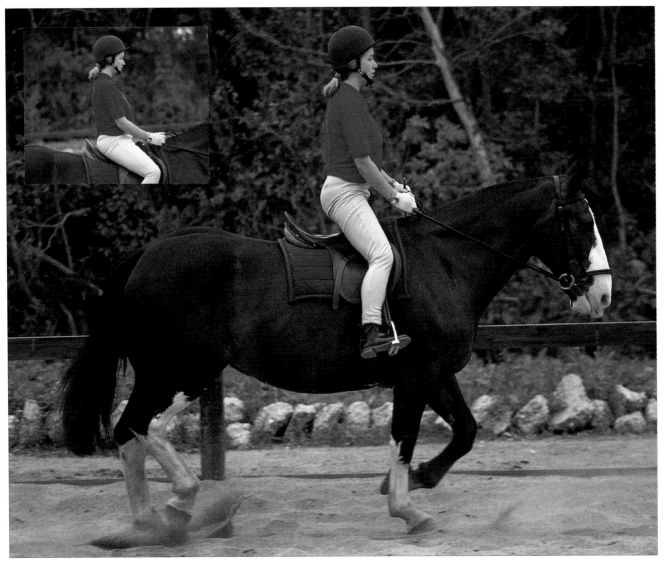

Cycling

Many cyclists suffer from neck, shoulder and back problems. This is because they often hunch over the handlebars, causing them to forcefully pull their head back to see where they are going. This is especially true of racing in competitions where dropped handlebars are often used, but it can also result from the incorrect adjustment of the saddle and handlebars, causing the cyclist to tense just to reach the pedals, for example.

Cycling can be a very enjoyable and beneficial sport, but often the cyclist's endeavour to become faster and faster stresses his or her body to a point where the muscles and joints become damaged; this damage may not become apparent until later on in life. With some thought about how you use your body while cycling, you will be able to ride more efficiently without placing your body under the enormous strain that is so common in the sport today. You need to be aware of your position so that you can consciously direct your body and help it to release any tension that may have accumulated.

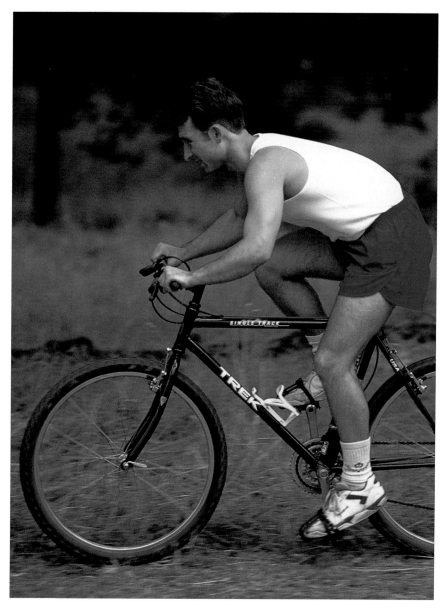

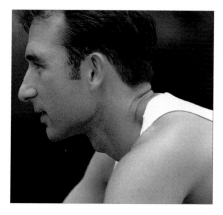

Above. *This cyclist endures severe neck tension as he endeavours to win the race – you can also see the strain in his jaw and facial muscles. He is so goal-orientated that he does not give any thought to how he is using his body. Aches and pains throughout his muscular system may result if this tension is allowed to persist, which could eventually force him to give up cycling altogether.*

Left. *This cyclist is leaning forward and down in an attempt to be more aerodynamic, yet his head is pulled back so that he can see where he is going. This places his neck and spine under enormous strain, which is likely to cause aches and pains in the upper part of the spine. If he cycles regularly in this position it is likely that this habit will be present even when he is not cycling.*

Right. *By having Alexander lessons you will be able to release the tension throughout the body and free the joints, thereby achieving a greater freedom of movement. Your teacher may also advise you to change the height of the saddle and handlebars; people often place unnecessary stress on their bodies simply because they have not correctly adjusted their bicycle to suit their needs.*

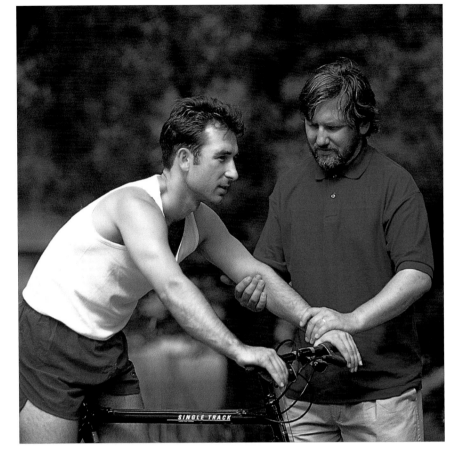

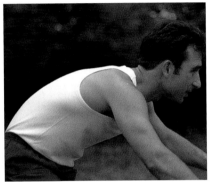

Above. *The position that this cyclist has adopted forces him to round his back, and if he continually cycles in this manner it is likely that he will begin to suffer from spinal problems.*

Right. *After having lessons both on and off the cycle track you will find that you use much less effort while cycling and achieve better results. This cyclist is now riding completely differently – his back is much straighter and his head is releasing forward and up away from his spine.*

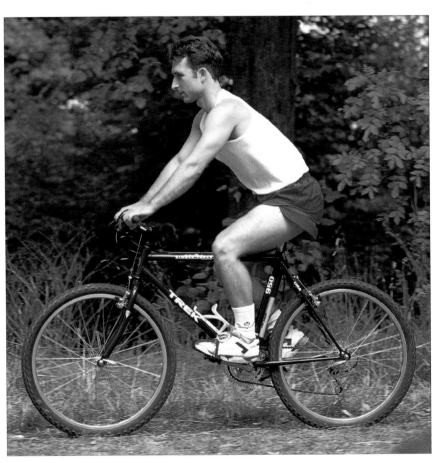

Running

Running is a very popular sport these days with many runners pushing themselves to the limit to become quicker or to run further. However, many of them give little thought to how they move and it is easy to see peculiar mannerisms when they run: feet spread out, chest raised, heels pulled back and tense arms and shoulders. The awkward ways of running adopted by many people are bound to create muscular tensions which can sometimes result in injuries: the over-tightened muscles produce sprains or muscle spasms, and later in life the person may develop arthritis of the hip, knee and ankle joints in particular ('runner's knee' is a common problem, for example). If runners push themselves too hard, they may find that they begin to suffer from backache, neckache or even more serious conditions in extreme cases.

With the grace and poise that can be obtained through practising the Alexander Technique, running can become a joy in itself, rather than a type of endurance test, which is how it has come to be viewed by many people. Out of all the sports, running is probably the most natural, as it exercises all the muscles of the body, and when the tension that competition brings is eliminated, the sensation of feeling your whole body moving freely and fluidly will remind you why you took up running in the first place.

Right. *This runner is actually leaning backwards with the effect that she is slowing herself down. She is totally unaware that she is doing this and would probably be very surprised if she saw this photograph of herself. Her arms now have to tense in order for her to keep her balance, and she is exaggerating her arm movements to help propel herself forward.*

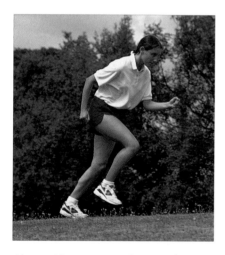

Above. *This runner is leaning forward and down, and as a result she is not looking where she is going. Her spine therefore has little chance of acting as the support for her body, so the muscles that should be free for movement are actually in tension.*

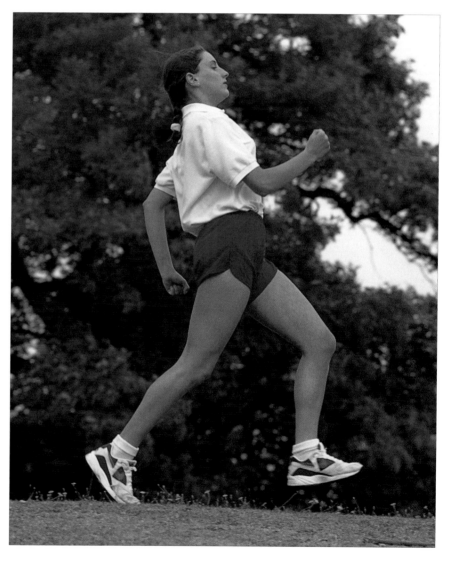

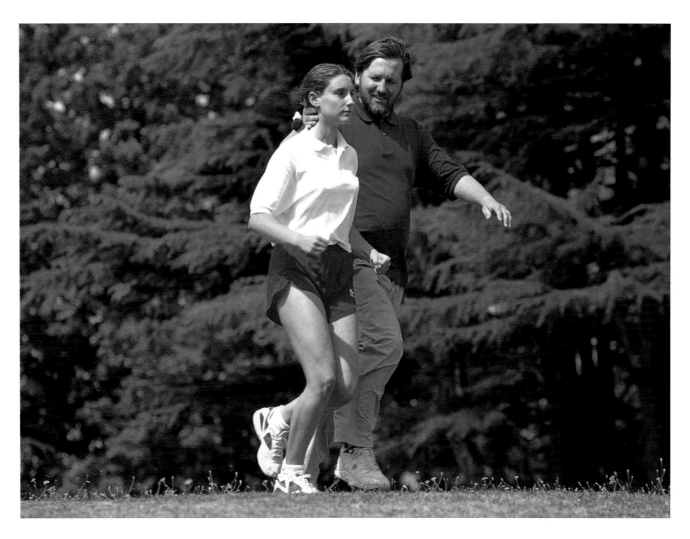

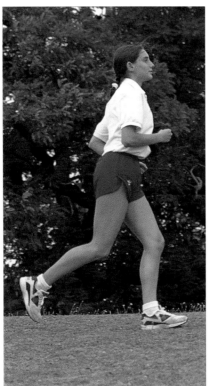 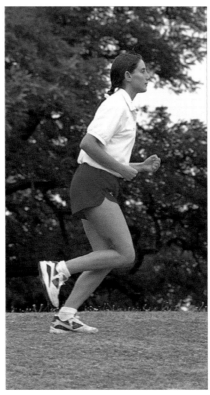

Above. *The Alexander Technique teacher is preventing her head from pulling backwards and as a result her spine is allowed to elongate. This allows her entire body to go forward and upwards into the run.*

Far left and left. *After some time you will be able to capture the feeling of freedom for yourself – not only will you be able to run more quickly and for longer periods, but your running will take on a new dimension. You may feel like all your joints have been oiled and you will move with a new sense of freedom and joy that you may not have felt since childhood. This runner's posture is now more upright: the spine is supporting the head, and the torso, arms and shoulders are now free to move fluidly. Her running is more graceful as a result, and she may even find that her speed improves without any effort on her part.*

93

Pool

Playing pool or snooker can also cause problems, although it is less stressful than many sports. Some of the positions that players have to adopt can put the body under an excessive amount of strain as they have to stretch or bend down to reach the ball. By being able to lengthen the muscles, it will give players new ways of releasing tension as they play their shots. Their game is likely to become more accurate as they will be more aware of the positions that cause tension within the body.

The main problem when playing pool or snooker is the backward retraction of the head which can often interfere with the primary control of the body. This has the effect of causing faulty sensory perception of the amount of muscular tension throughout the body, which in turn prevents the fluidity of movement in the joints that is required for a successful game. Many snooker and pool players are amazed to find how much more accurate their shots are once they have released the muscular tension of which they were previously unaware.

Right. *This is a typical stance that many players adopt. The legs are braced backwards causing the spine to bend, which puts a great strain on the back muscles.*

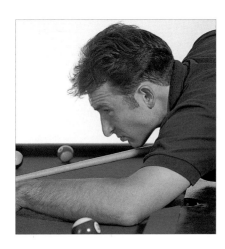

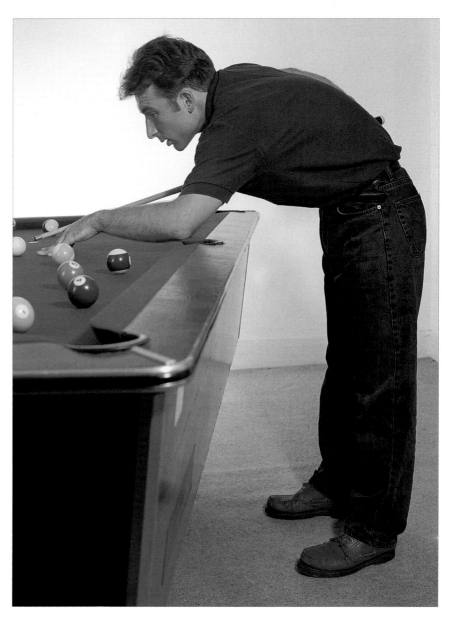

Above. *A close look at the head and shoulders reveals that the head is pulling backwards with a great force, compressing many of the intervertebral discs. If this position is adopted regularly it could lead to neck and back problems in later life. This tension can also cause inaccurate shots because the shoulders and arms are not able to move freely.*

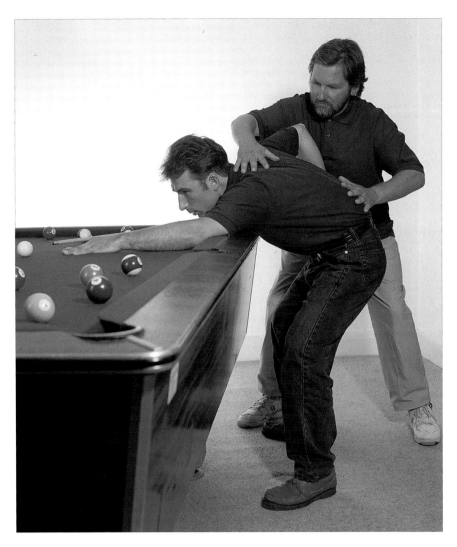

Left. *By lengthening the back and allowing the knees to bend, the player learns new ways of bending which put less strain on the muscular and skeletal systems. Consequently, the neck muscles also become less tense, which affects the relationship of the head, neck and back. By bending at the knee, ankle and hip joints the spinal curves are less exaggerated, and as a result there is not so much force pulling the head back.*

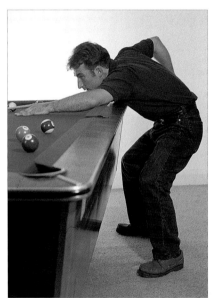

Above. *After a while the player becomes used to this new way of playing. Now it is the hip, knee and ankle joints that take him lower and keep his spine lengthened, so reducing the harmful tension in his neck.*

Left. *Placing one foot behind the other gives more support to the rest of the body and allows a greater freedom of movement. As a result, there is likely to be a dramatic improvement in the player's game as he is now able to play his shots with greater accuracy.*

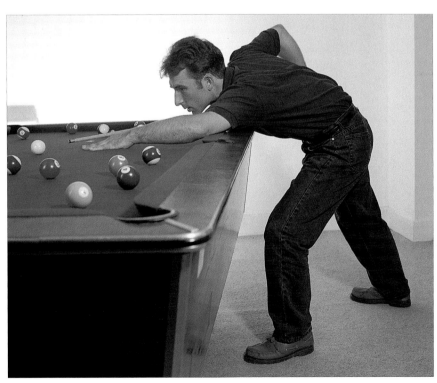

95

Tennis

Alexander Technique lessons will not replace your need for tennis coaching, but by having help to release muscle tension you will find that your body can respond more easily and quickly, which will naturally improve your play. You will be more aware of over-gripping your racket – this can cause you to mishit shots or can cause muscle tension in the wrist, elbow and arm muscles. This over-gripping of the racket, or using your wrist incorrectly in certain strokes, particularly the backhand, is usually responsible for 'tennis elbow'. Tennis

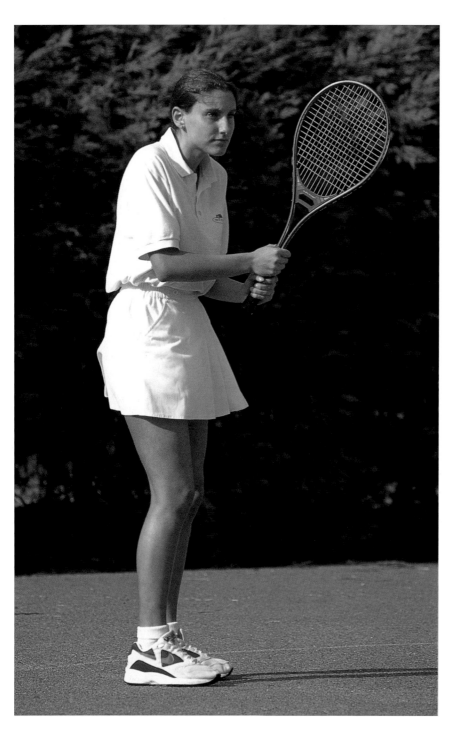

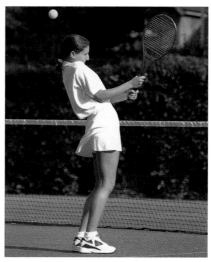

Left. *This woman is so concentrated on what her opponent is doing that she is unaware that she is in an inappropriate position to receive the ball. Her knees should be bent and she should be on her toes, ready to move in any direction. Notice how she is tensing her neck muscles in her effort to achieve success.*

Above. *When the ball is returned she is caught off balance and as a result her muscular system is more concerned with keeping her upright than with getting the ball back over the net. This creates tension particularly in the neck, back and legs. The result will nearly always be failure to do what she knows she is capable of and, if she continually plays under such strain, it could result in her losing the game altogether.*

Right. *Here the teacher is getting the primary control (the dynamic relationship of the head with the neck and back) to respond as it should. The tennis player's whole body will then be freer, and she will be able to adopt a suitable position from which to return the ball more easily.*

Below. *Her hands are gripping the tennis racket with much more tension than is necessary. This will result in her mishitting the ball or striking it with too much force, so that it frequently goes out of play. Just by being aware of how you are holding your racket will automatically improve your grip – your hands will become more relaxed as the tension in your fingers and wrists releases.*

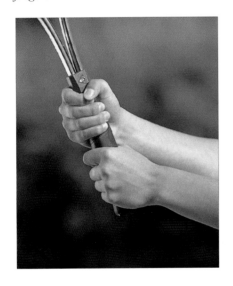

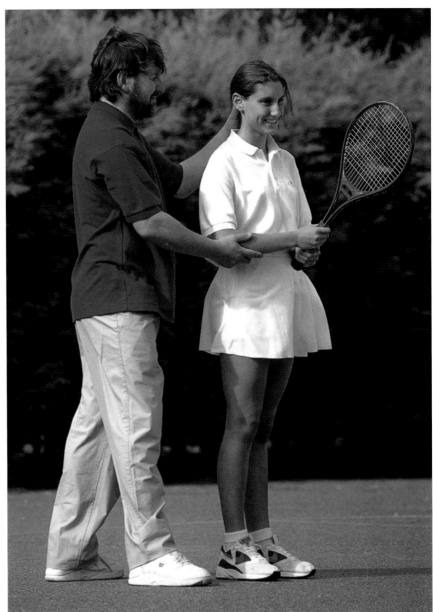

elbow causes pain on the outer side of the elbow, and the pain can become more severe on certain movements.

By pausing before you act it will help you to feel that you have more time to react positively to the approaching ball, as you will be less likely to rush and misread your opponent's shot. Although it will often seem as though there is no time to think before you hit the ball, all you need to do is to take a moment to be aware of your actions so that you can consciously direct yourself before you play the shot. The more you are able to release your muscular system, the more fluid your shots will be and you will find that you

are easily reaching shots that you might previously have missed *(see also overleaf)*. It is also very important to be aware of your stance when you are waiting for your opponent to return the ball. You should be bent at the knee and hip joints and your whole body should be in balance. Alexander referred to this as the 'position of mechanical advantage', as your body can respond more quickly since it is in a state of alertness. And you will be more prepared for the spin that your opponent may put on the ball.

Your increased confidence in your own playing ability will also play an important psychological part in winning the game.

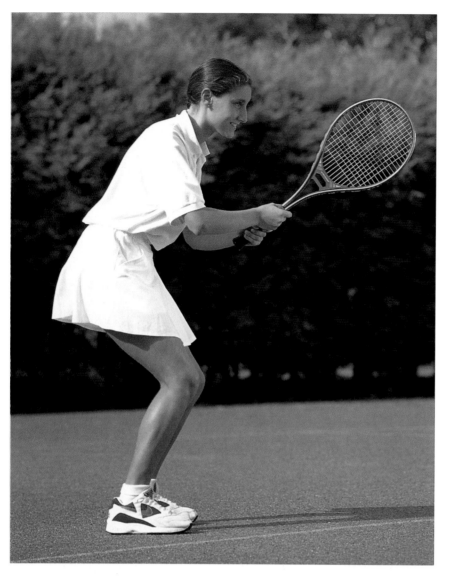

Left. *This is the best stance to adopt when getting ready for your opponent's serve. A slightly squatting stance (Alexander called it the 'position of mechanical advantage') increases the range of movements possible when returning the ball. It also promotes alertness. Notice how her head is in alignment with her spine and her shoulders are not hunched over, allowing her the freedom of movement to return the serve to the maximum of her ability.*

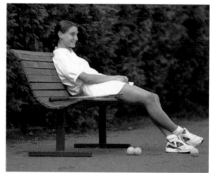

Above. *Even the way you sit between games can affect your play – sitting like this can make you feel tired or lethargic when you return to the court, because your body is not getting the rest it needs. Her back is rounded and is under stress, and consequently she has to push her head and neck forward to see what is going on around her.*

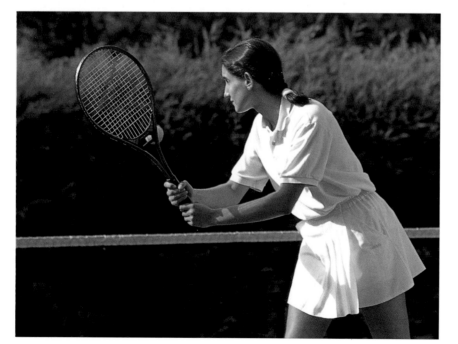

Left. *By thinking of her head leading and her back lengthening, she will be more agile and therefore likely to reach shots that she would previously have missed. She will also be able to achieve a smooth flow of play more easily and not become so frustrated when she misses a shot.*

Don't be hard on yourself

Success comes when your mind is at peace and your inner critic is not telling you to do better or punishing you for the mistake you made five minutes ago. The moments when any sport feels the most rewarding are when little effort is required for even the most demanding of actions, and you just feel a natural flow that helps you to excel your usual performance. This, in turn, gives you more confidence to perform the next movement effortlessly. This spontaneous state is hard to achieve, yet it is possible to cultivate the feeling if only we stop trying so hard and 'let it happen'. In the foreword to Eugen Herrigel's book *Zen in the Art of Archery*, D. T. Suzuki describes the effects of a busy mind on archery:

> *'As soon as we reflect, deliberate, and conceptualize, the original unconscious is lost and a thought interferes … Man is a thinking reed but his great works are done when he is not calculating and thinking.'*

Many people are involved in sport to achieve a heightened state of awareness rather than to win trophies (except, perhaps, professional sportspeople!). No matter what your sport, there can be a point during the activity when you reach a stillness, your over-active mind becomes calm and the only place is 'here' and the time is 'now' – nothing exists outside that present moment. You reach a point where an indescribable feeling of oneness takes place: the runner becomes merged with the elements; the tennis player feels that the racket is merely an extension of his or her own arm; the rider and the horse become so interconnected that they move as one entity; the surfer maintains the correct poise and delicate balance to negotiate the power of the waves; and the skier is taken down the slope at incredible speeds and performs the perfect action at precisely the right moment without thought or effort. In this state of mind your inner critic is silenced and you no longer care whether you are winning or losing – you are simply experiencing a feeling of joy and total connection with the present moment. The Alexander Technique helps you to be aware of the habits that stop this perfect flow from taking place, and through gradual non-interference we can allow that feeling to manifest.

The same principles apply to the less active games, such as chess or the ancient oriental game of Go, where the true triumph over obstacles takes place in the players' minds rather than on the board. In both games, success is achieved when inhibition is exercised and panic and 'end-gaining' are eliminated; it is only then that inner peace prevails and the true excellence of the player can be revealed.

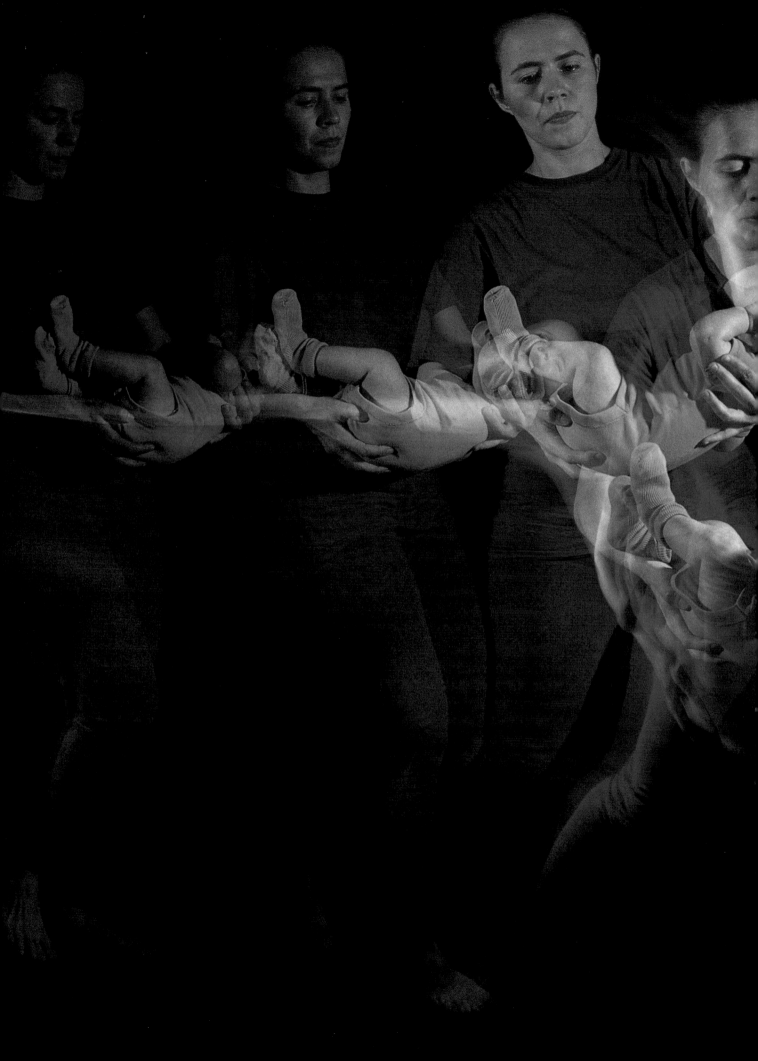

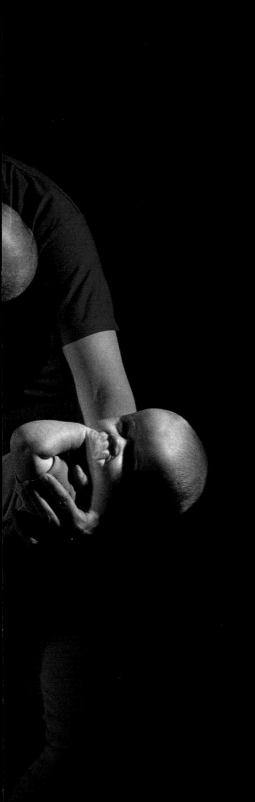

CHAPTER SEVEN

Pregnancy and childbirth

'The more a woman accomplishes in her feminine, natural functions knowingly and wilfully, particularly in labour, in the birth of her infant, and in its nourishment, the more she learns, both intuitively and consciously. The more she appreciates herself in so doing, the more her self-appreciation radiates towards her infant and others – her husband, her other children, and society.'

Dr William Hazlett

The Alexander Technique teaches you how to lift and carry your child without placing your joints and muscles under excessive strain, so helping you to avoid neck and back problems. Your baby will also benefit from your increased ease and receptivity to his or her needs, and this will result in your baby being more content.

Pregnancy and childbirth

A far more specialized application of the Alexander Technique is during pregnancy and childbirth. Many people do not realize that the Technique can be invaluable at this time of life, and can be practised throughout pregnancy, childbirth and even when caring for your baby afterwards. The harmful postural habits many women have adopted, such as leaning backwards by pushing their hips forward and arching their back, and consequently poking their head forwards, are often exacerbated during pregnancy, and this can easily be seen in the way they sit and stand. The postures they tend to adopt often result in chronic back pain and general fatigue, much of which could be avoided by having Alexander lessons.

Apart from the physical aspects with which the Technique can help, there are other, less obvious but equally important, issues about making conscious and informed choices throughout the pregnancy, as well as during and after the birth of the child. Yet it is common in our society for many of these decisions to be taken out of the hands of the parents as a matter of course. Alexander primarily saw his Technique as the key to enabling a person to exercise real choice in his or her life, and there are many crucial decisions to be made during this very important time.

It is also important to realize that each woman may have very different experiences in pregnancy and especially during labour, and there are very few formulae you can follow to achieve the 'perfect birth'. The secret is to be ready for anything, because the power of nature is a very formidable and unpredictable force, and once the process has started it is much easier to work with it than against it.

Pregnancy

Some midwives say that they can often predict whether the labour is going to be difficult or easy by the general attitude of the mother-to-be: the more relaxed and easy-going she is, the more likely it is that she will experience an uncomplicated birth. By having Alexander lessons during or immediately preceding pregnancy you will be more prepared, both physically and mentally, for one of the most incredible experiences of your life. If you do suffer from anxiety or tension you may find that the Technique helps enormously in letting go of your fear and apprehension about the birth and motherhood itself. Your heightened awareness of your body, both physically and emotionally, and the fact that your body is naturally undergoing enormous and rapid alterations, aid the process of change that the Alexander Technique aims to bring about. You will be able to comprehend and let go of unwanted habits more easily at this time in your life than perhaps at any other.

The gain in weight of your unborn baby, the placenta and the amniotic fluid (the protective fluid surrounding the growing foetus) will be about 5.5 kg (12 lb), but the overall increase may be two or even three times this figure. This will vary from woman to woman, but the average increase in weight during pregnancy is a staggering 12.5 kg (27½ lb). This will obviously have a dramatic effect on the way you move, sit and stand, and unconscious habits will often become magnified during pregnancy due to the additional strain your body is under.

A common example of this can be seen in the tendency to lean back while standing; pregnant women are often quite oblivious to the fact that they are arching their back and pushing their hips forward, which results in an imbalance and strain affecting their entire body. The increase in weight of the womb will result in this habit being exaggerated, causing the lower spine to be compressed and increasing the likelihood of severe backache. This swaying back is so common in our Western society that many women suffer unnecessarily from chronic backache during pregnancy.

With the extra weight of the developing foetus, many of the muscles in the front of the body are put under more strain, causing them to shorten and often resulting in a 'pulling down' sensation. To compensate for this feeling, many women tend to arch their lumbar curve, which then leads to the entire body being out of balance. During your lessons you will be taught how to release this muscle tension, giving you a sensation of lengthening and releasing both the front and back muscles. You may even become taller as your spine lengthens as well as strengthens, which can help to support your baby with less effort. After a number of lessons these muscles will be more effective in supporting the extra

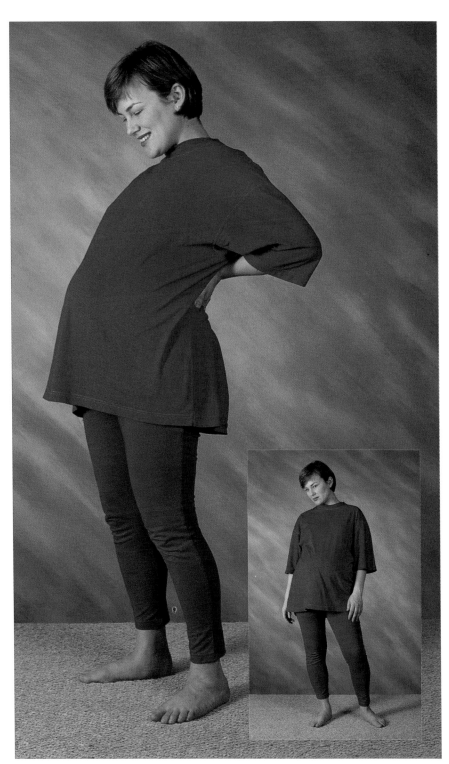

Left. *Backache is very common, especially in the last few months of pregnancy. As the baby grows there is more weight in front and most women compensate by leaning backwards; this pushes the pelvis forward and arches the lumbar spine. Excess tension in the back is responsible for the faulty sensory perception of standing up straight.*

Inset. *To help alleviate back pain it is common for pregnant women to sink down on to one hip which only brings temporary relief and adversely affects their body alignment. This stance puts too much pressure on the hip joint and causes a general over-tightening of the muscular system, as well as probably resulting in backache.*

Below. *Even at rest it is common for many pregnant women to slump when sitting, which further aggravates their backache. When in pain they are likely to tense up all their muscles and this can affect their baby's movement. This woman is trying to get comfortable by leaning back on the chair, but this position does not allow her spine to act as a supportive structure to her body. She is also pushing her neck forward, causing tension in the neck muscles.*

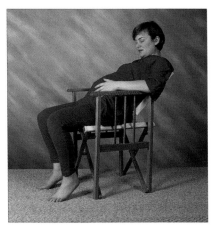

Right. *Alexander Technique lessons will help you to move in a different way so that you will feel as comfortable as possible during your pregnancy. Here, the teacher is helping this woman to lengthen and widen her back so that the muscles do not have to do so much work. This produces a feeling of lightness in her body, and helps her to move with greater ease.*

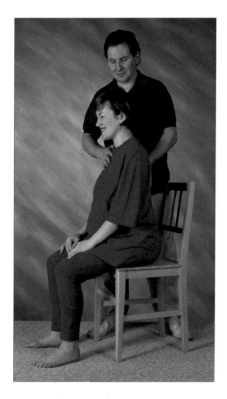

Above. *The entire balance and centre of gravity of your body is being constantly readjusted as your baby increases in size. With the help of an Alexander teacher, you will be able to readjust your balance to accommodate the extra weight, thereby minimizing the strain on your body. Here, the teacher is helping the woman to lengthen the muscles in the front of her body so that her spine becomes straighter and is therefore more aligned to carry the weight of the head.*

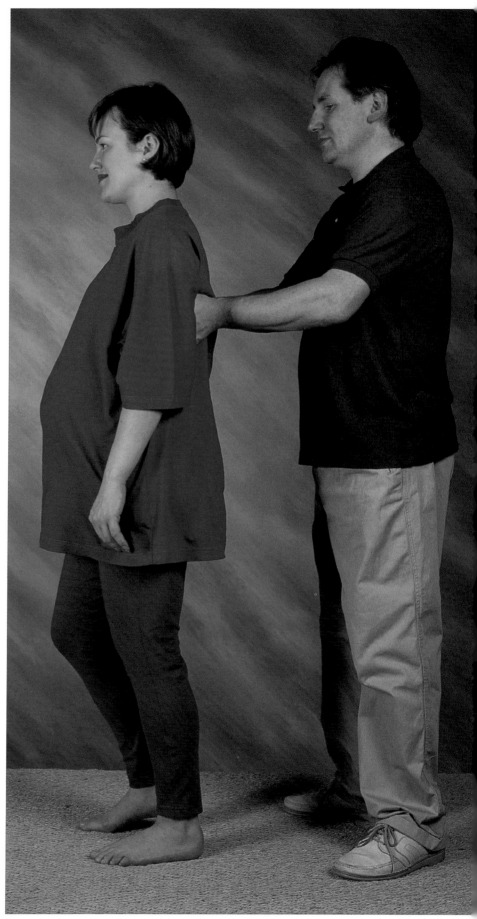

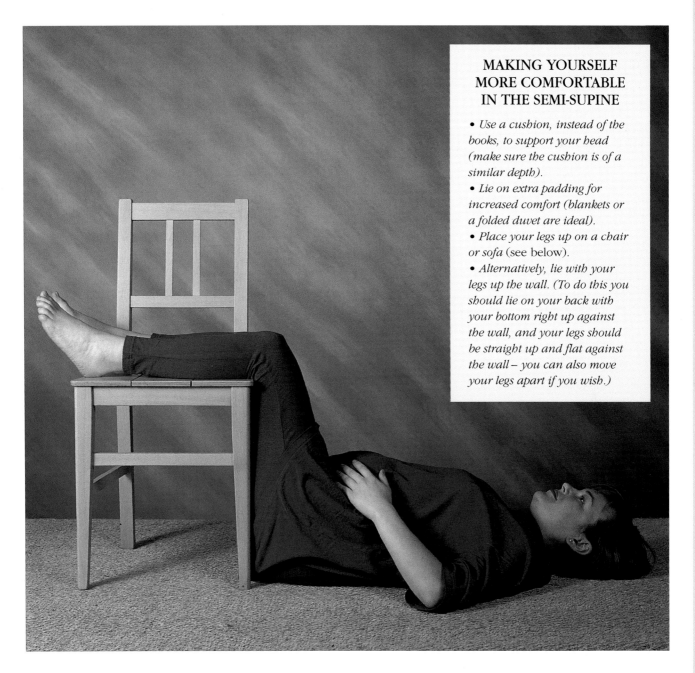

**MAKING YOURSELF
MORE COMFORTABLE
IN THE SEMI-SUPINE**

• *Use a cushion, instead of the
books, to support your head
(make sure the cushion is of a
similar depth).*
• *Lie on extra padding for
increased comfort (blankets or
a folded duvet are ideal).*
• *Place your legs up on a chair
or sofa (see below).*
• *Alternatively, lie with your
legs up the wall. (To do this you
should lie on your back with
your bottom right up against
the wall, and your legs should
be straight up and flat against
the wall – you can also move
your legs apart if you wish.)*

weight of the developing womb, giving you a
feeling of increased lightness and ease. The
increased comfort that you will experience as
you go about your daily activities will give
you a greater sense of well-being, and this will
help you to cope with the enormous mental
and emotional changes that are taking place.

*A good resting position during your pregnancy is to lie on
your back with your legs on a chair. This will relieve
backache and any tension that has built up in the pelvic
area, as it eases the downward pressure of the baby.*

Resting positions

During your pregnancy it is essential that you
rest your body as much as possible, even in
the early months as this is when miscarriages
are more common. For the first few months
you will find it very helpful to lie down in the
semi-supine position as described in chapter
five *(see page 70)*, as this is one of the best
resting positions for your body. It encourages
your spine to lengthen, as well as relaxing
over-tense muscles. This will give your baby
more room in which to grow, as well as helping you to have a greater capacity for breathing more deeply, which can often enhance
a feeling of peace and contentment. As the

pregnancy progresses, however, there are certain steps you can follow to achieve extra comfort when lying down in the semi-supine position *(see previous page)*.

There may come a time in the later stages of pregnancy when lying on your back will start to become uncomfortable or even painful. Do *not* persevere – it is the body's way of saying that this is no longer appropriate. Lying on your side with your knees bent may be of some help at this stage. When lying down in the semi-supine position during the last three months of your pregnancy there is a possibility that the weight of your baby may compress the inferior vena cava, one of the major blood vessels that carries the blood from the legs back to the heart. Sometimes this

can reduce the blood flow to the placenta, and if this happens you will start to feel faint or nauseous, so it is better to avoid the semi-supine position in the last three months. *Remember:* listen to your body – it knows best.

How the body changes

There are two other important occurrences which take place during pregnancy. The first is the releasing of the hormones progesterone and relaxin from the placenta, which naturally causes the connective tissues and ligaments in the body to become more elastic. This allows the joints of the spine and pelvis to become more flexible in preparation for the birth. The second is the enormous increase in fluid content within body tissues, causing the muscles

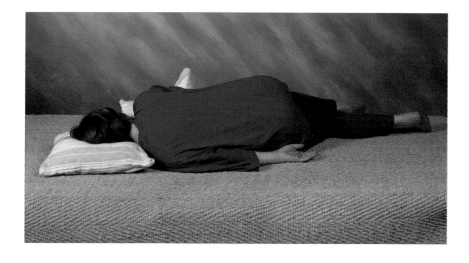

Right and below. *This is another good resting position that you might find more comfortable as your pregnancy progresses. Using pillows to support your head and leg, you can still think of releasing tension by allowing your back to lengthen and widen. You may also wish to use this position when sleeping.*

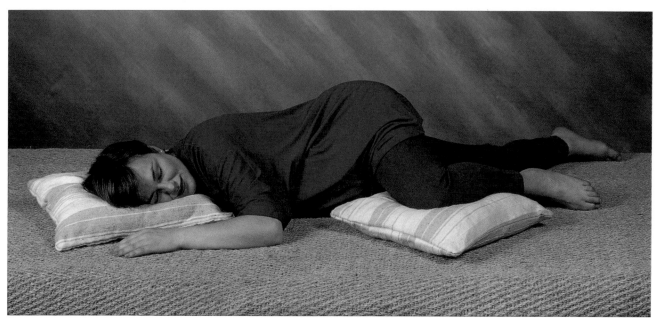

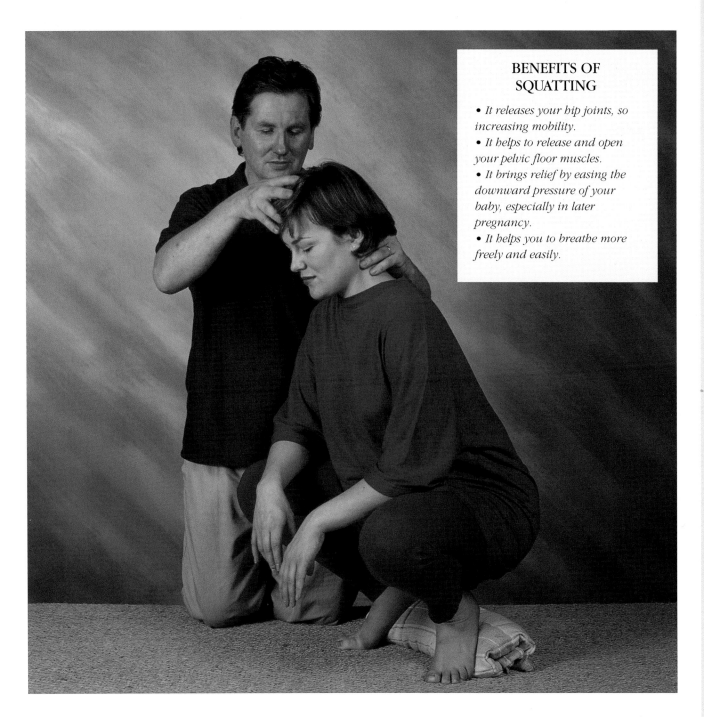

BENEFITS OF SQUATTING

- *It releases your hip joints, so increasing mobility.*
- *It helps to release and open your pelvic floor muscles.*
- *It brings relief by easing the downward pressure of your baby, especially in later pregnancy.*
- *It helps you to breathe more freely and easily.*

to become more pliable. Due to these changes your body becomes much more flexible, and many women find that their body is much more supple than usual (which is another reason why Alexander lessons during pregnancy can often have a greater effect than at any other time in your life). You also need to be aware that owing to these natural changes to the body's systems you will be more vulnerable to injury and need to take greater care not to stress your body, especially at work or by doing strenuous exercises.

Your Alexander Technique teacher will gently take you through movements like squatting that will be beneficial during your pregnancy and labour so that you do not over-strain yourself when you do them on your own. You may find it helpful to place a cushion behind your feet so that you feel more balanced. The teacher is making sure that this woman keeps her neck free and keeps her head going forward and up so that her spine can lengthen.

The benefits of squatting

Squatting is another useful position to practise during pregnancy, in preparation for your

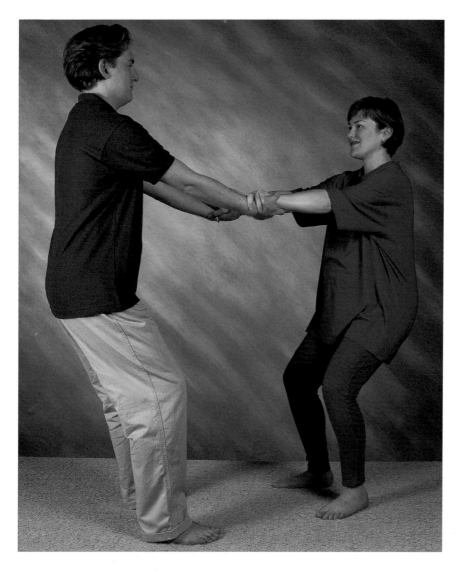

Left and below. *Squatting with your partner or using a chair for support throughout your pregnancy can help the pelvic floor muscles to release. These are the muscles that often tear during labour, so by releasing them you minimize the chances of this happening. Squatting during labour can also help you to have an easier and quicker birth.*

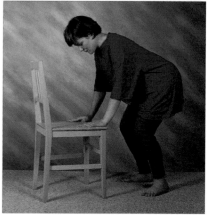

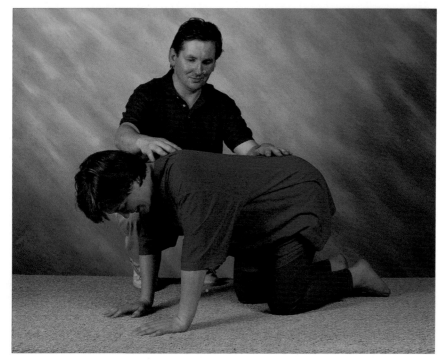

Left. *During your lessons you will also be shown how to get the most out of various resting positions that help to release tension and strengthen the back, so that you will be well prepared for your labour. Here, the teacher is helping the woman to lengthen her whole spine so that it can support the body's weight more effectively.*

labour. In this position your pelvis is opened to its widest extent and the downward force of gravity will aid the birth process, but it also has other benefits during the pregnancy.

If you find a full squat difficult then try the more shallow type *(see opposite)*, making sure you do not strain yourself in the process; the deeper squats will get easier with practice.

Due to the additional elasticity of the muscles, you will find that you can bend with greater ease, and your Alexander teacher will help you to move in and out of the squat as effortlessly as possible. You will also be helped to achieve equilibrium while squatting, which is essential for comfort and the elimination of muscle strain. It is a good idea

to practise squatting as a natural part of your everyday activities, so that when it comes to the labour you will be able to maintain the position more easily.

Exercises at home

Most teachers of the Alexander Technique do not advocate certain physical exercises as they only make a habit more ingrained. However, natural movements like walking, running and swimming are beneficial as they exercise the whole body rather than just certain muscles in particular. There are a number of pre-natal exercises that you can practise safely at home *(see below and overleaf)*, and if you apply your directions and release tension as you do these

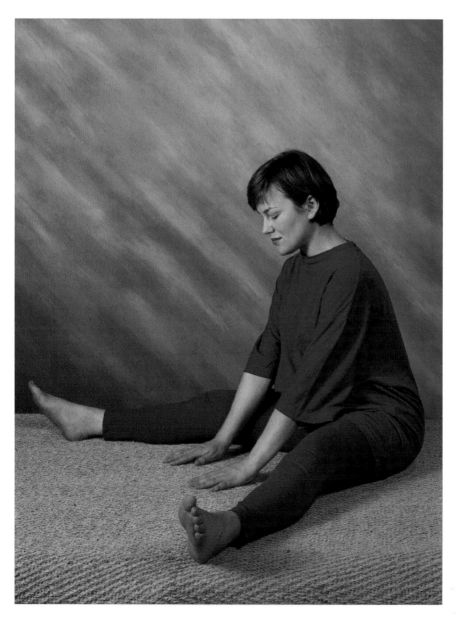

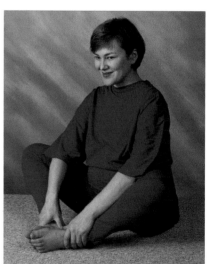

Left. *This position helps to release tension in the inner thigh muscles. Sit with your legs far apart, without straining, and then think of your inner thighs lengthening away from each other. The lengthening of these muscles can help you to give birth more easily.*

Above. *This is another common posture that helps to release the pelvic floor muscles. Be careful not to force your legs apart; instead you could think of letting your legs release away from one another, which again will lengthen the inner thighs. If you allow the soles of your feet to touch it will help you to release the inner thigh muscles more effectively. Make sure that your back does not slump while sitting in this position.*

Below. *It is common for pregnant women to compensate for the extra weight of the baby by swaying back from the pelvis. Stand side on to a mirror and raise both arms up in front of you – check to see if you are arching your back and throwing your hips forward in a way similar to this woman.*

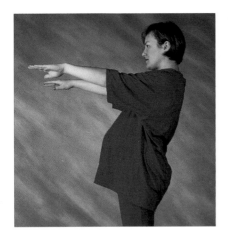

Right. *Do the same exercise, but this time when you raise your arms compensate for the weight change by slightly leaning back from the ankle joints and keeping your back straight. This will help you to learn to compensate for the extra weight you are carrying as you go about your day-to-day activities. If you can be aware of this in later pregnancy as your baby develops, you will avoid much of the backache that many woman take for granted during the last months of pregnancy.*

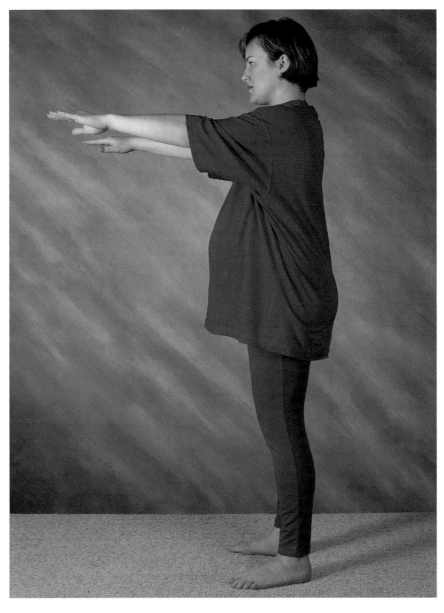

exercises, it will be far more beneficial than forcing your muscles to stretch.

Breathing

Alexander re-education can be invaluable here. There are a number of ideas and theories on varying breathing techniques to adopt during pregnancy and labour, and while some may be helpful in certain circumstances during labour, most tend to interfere with the normal respiratory process. The main thing you can do to help your body throughout pregnancy and labour is to be more aware of your breath and allow yourself to finish one breath before you start another. It is surprising how many adults have forgotten how to breathe freely: habits of snatching or holding breath during times of anxiety and stress are very common.

During your pregnancy it is very useful to practise 'the whispered ah' as described in chapter four *(see page 56)*. Vocalized 'ah' sounds while relaxing the jaw and other facial muscles can also be very beneficial. The secret is always to focus on the out-breath, as this determines the intake of air. It is a good idea to spend a few minutes each day breathing in this way so that when your labour starts it will be very familiar to you and therefore can be done without too much concentration.

You must not forget that you are breathing for two (or perhaps more!) and there will be changes in your pattern of breathing to cope with this. Your growing baby will gradually take up more and more space, giving your lungs and other organs less room in which to function. This will cause an increase in your respiration rate and you will find that you may become more breathless during activities such as ascending stairs. Try to be aware of your breath as you allow the in-breath to expand both downward and outward, so that the maximum amount of air is taken in without straining. It is important that you do not rush any of these breathing techniques, as this can interfere detrimentally with your breathing itself, so defeating the purpose of practising the techniques in the first place.

Making choices

There is much controversy over whether home or hospital births provide a safer environment, but when all is said and done it is your birth and therefore has to be your decision. This freedom to choose what is best for *you* is at the very heart of the Alexander Technique. One of the first decisions you will have to make once you know you are pregnant is whether you want to have your baby in hospital or at home, but no matter what you decide do not forget that you always have the right to change your mind, even at the last moment. For the mother, the act of bearing a child, and for the father, seeing your own child being born, can be one of the most moving and beautiful experiences of one's life, but if you are not prepared it can sometimes be quite a terrifying one. This is why it is crucial for you to make your decisions before the labour starts, as this can often make all the difference.

Whether the birth takes place in hospital or at home, it is important to have a birth plan that you have decided upon *before* labour begins. Make sure anyone present at the birth knows of your wishes – the last thing you need during your labour is the frustration of trying to communicate to the midwife or doctor between contractions what you do or do not want! The two different environments – hospital and home – can provide very different

experiences for both mother and child, and each has its own advantages and drawbacks. There are a number of books you can refer to in order to make an informed choice *(see 'further reading' on page 141)* – but remember, you should choose what is best for *you*.

You may think that some of these issues seem to have nothing to do with the Alexander Technique, but in my view the mother is consciously making an informed choice whether or not to interfere with the natural processes of giving birth. The principles of not interfering with nature, increased awareness and exercising free choice are all at the heart of the Alexander Technique.

Childbirth

This is often the most unpredictable part of the pregnancy, for no two labours are the same – not even for the same woman. The secret is to be as prepared as possible without having any expectations; this may sound like a contradiction in terms, but there is a fine line between the two.

As the labour progresses, you may find it hard to recall mentally what you have learned during your Alexander lessons about inhibiting, thinking of your directions and releasing tension, but do not worry because the preparation you have done during your pregnancy will benefit you now. Your body will remember what to do at a very deep instinctual level; all you can hope to do is not to interfere consciously with the powerful process that is taking place. You must forget about everyone around you and make sure that you do not try to please anyone but yourself, despite the fact that this sometimes goes against life-long habits and conditioning about politeness and selfishness.

There are many books and people (both qualified and unqualified) who will offer you conflicting advice, and, while it may be important to listen to some of them it is vital that you make your own conscious choice about the sort of labour you want, based on your own powerful instincts and intuition. As with other matters, human beings are inclined to interfere unnecessarily with what is essentially a perfectly natural process, and while it is very reassuring to know that certain drugs and procedures can ensure the mother and baby's safety, it is also important to be aware that the very same drugs and procedures can sometimes cause complications during the birth.

Labour

The best way to deal with labour is to trust the process and try to let go of any preconceived ideas of how it should proceed. Even the birth plan may have to go by the board in certain situations. Just stay with your breath as much as you are able.

The first stage

This stage usually begins with the onset of regular contractions or the waters breaking, and ends when the cervix is fully dilated. It is extremely difficult to predict how long this phase will last and how uncomfortable it will be. It can take only two or three hours, or it might last for more than a day.

Right. *The knee-to-chest position is a very useful resting position that you may want to adopt between contractions. It has the advantage of slowing the labour down if the process is progressing too quickly and you are beginning to feel out of control, and it can also help to lengthen the back and neck.*

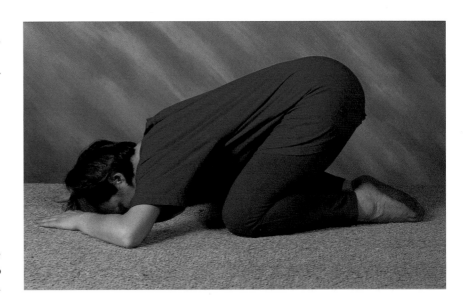

Below. *This resting position helps to maintain a lengthened spine and encourages the stomach muscles to relax between contractions. Your muscular system will be able to release tension more effectively in this position because your body has more support. It can also be a good position in which to give birth.*

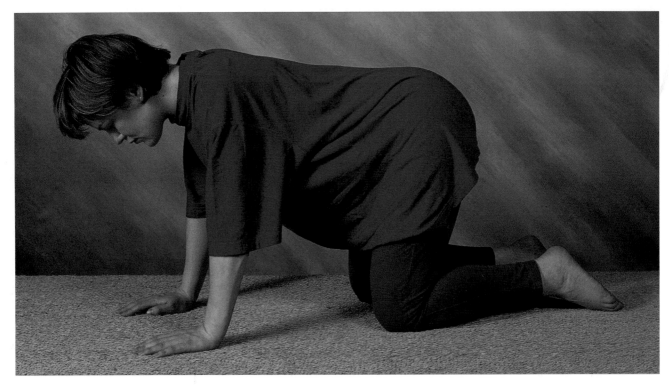

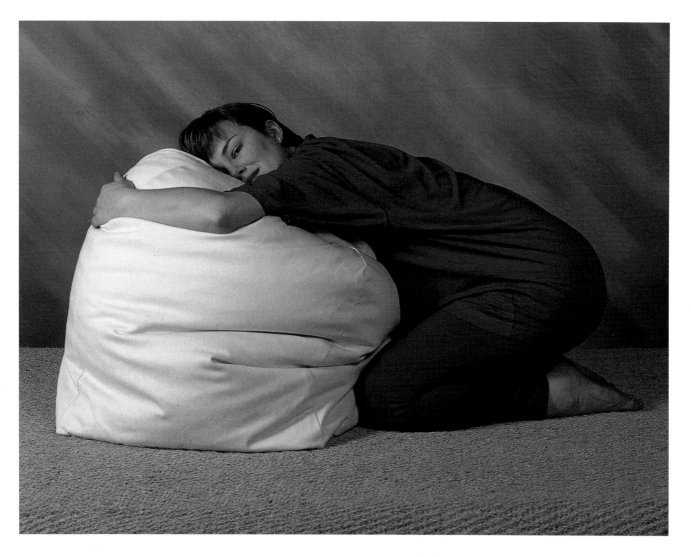

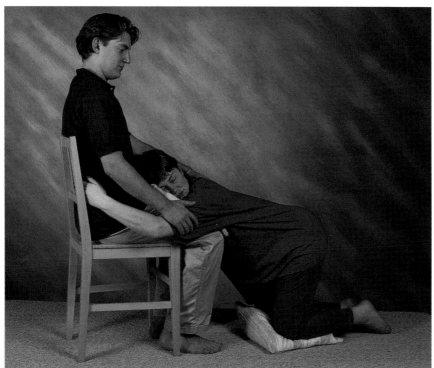

Above and left. *These are good resting positions to adopt throughout your pregnancy, but they can also be used between contractions, as they allow your body to be supported and encourage the stomach muscles to release. You may find that resting your head in your partner's lap helps to make you feel more relaxed. You can also use this position to give birth as an alternative to squatting.*

113

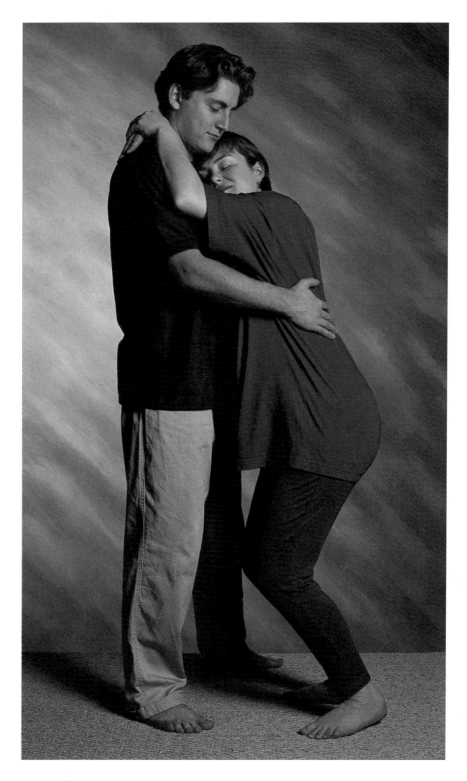

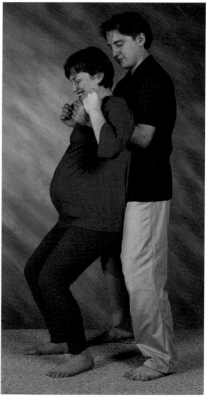

Left. Squatting during labour is an extremely good position to be in – with the help of gravity the baby's head is pushed downwards and this speeds the process up by assisting the pelvic floor muscles to release. It may be helpful for you to have the support of your partner or midwife during this time.

Above. Being supported from behind can be very advantageous during the second stage of labour: the woman can stand without straining her muscles, and the more relaxed she is, the better it is for the birth itself. This is also an ideal position for giving birth, as the baby is again helped down the birth canal by gravity.

In the first stage your contractions will often start gently and build up until they are very intense, resulting in discomfort and pain. It is easy to tense against these contractions rather than letting them work. We naturally associate pain with something not being right, but this is the exception to the rule. It is worth remembering that pain in this case is perfectly natural. It is constructive, and part of the process that brings your baby into the world. The more you can go with the contractions rather than fight against them, the easier the birth you will have.

During this first stage of labour it is important to find a comfortable position to suit you, and most women instinctively choose to stand up or walk about – it is common for them to lean or hang on to a convenient object or their partner. When you are upright, the downward force of gravity will assist in your baby's descent and will stimulate contractions and the dilation of the cervix. There will be times when you will need to rest, and sitting on a low stool or on the edge of a chair with your legs apart while leaning forward can be very comfortable. This will also help to lengthen the spine which will give your body extra support, even if you are not conscious of it at the time. Some women find sitting on the toilet another very comfortable position.

During long labours there may be times when you wish to rest, and it may sometimes be appropriate to lie down on your side with some cushions to support your legs and head *(see page 106)*. Squatting can be very useful during this stage, especially if the labour is prolonged, as it can speed up the contractions. Lying down on your back during labour, however, is probably one of the worst positions to be in, as it hinders the birth process because the contractions now have to push the baby horizontally along the birth canal instead of downwards, where they are assisted by gravity. This will probably increase the length of the labour and may result in tearing, and is likely to make you feel too exhausted to push during the second stage. There is also the danger that the baby may exert pressure on to one of the main blood vessels, restricting the blood flow. In fact, the reason why many hospital births are carried out in this way is because it is easier for the doctors and midwives to assess the progress of the labour. Women may also have to lie down when they have oxytocin and epidural drips, or if they are wired up to equipment which monitors the contractions and the baby's pulse.

Transition

There is usually a definite transition period between the first and second stages. During this time your contractions may be at their most powerful, and there is often a sense of losing control – your movements may be wildly unpredictable. You might find that you feel like giving up, or that you would do anything to make the pain go away. It is also possible that there may be a lull in the contractions and you may be able to get some rest. Your Alexander lessons up to this point should help you to remain as calm as you can be in this situation; your body will have learned how to relax and release any unwanted tension, and it will instinctively remember what to do even though the Alexander Technique may be the last thing on your mind at this time!

The second stage

This stage starts when the cervix is fully dilated and ends with the birth of the baby; it can last anything from just a few minutes to a couple of hours. During this stage squatting is one of the most useful positions to adopt; after all, it is probable that women have given birth this way for as long as humans have roamed the earth. In less material societies, like India or Africa for example, squatting is an everyday activity, so when it comes to childbirth this position is adopted naturally. In Western societies many women can find squatting unaided very strenuous, and you may need to be supported by your partner or midwife *(see opposite),* or even both. If you have become accustomed to squatting during your pregnancy then you will be happier with this extremely beneficial stance. While you are squatting, not only does the force of gravity help to expel your baby, but the pelvic outlet is as much as 2 cm (¾ in) wider than in other positions.

When the baby's head can first be seen, another useful position is to kneel leaning forward over a chair or even to be on all fours – both these positions allow more time for the baby to be born. Although at this point you will probably feel as though you want to get the birth over with as quickly as possible, it will actually reduce the risk of tearing and avoid the possibility of a panic situation occurring, which can sometimes happen if the baby's body is born too fast. It is vital not to tense at this point, but to work with your breath: some women naturally find themselves wanting to scream or shout. This can actually aid the birth process, since it forces the abdomen to bear down.

The third stage

This stage starts from the moment your baby is born and ends with the expulsion of the placenta. If this is speeded up artificially by using the drug syntometrine (which is extremely common in Western hospitals), then it is best for you to lie down while the doctor or midwife removes the detached placenta. If this drug is used, the cord must be clamped and cut without delay. If you opt for the more natural method, then it is better for you to breastfeed your baby immediately, as this will help to speed up the retraction of the uterus, which naturally expels the placenta. It is an interesting fact that the umbilical cord is often long enough to be still attached during that first breastfeed.

It is, however, important to realize that some babies are not interested in feeding straight away, and this should not be forced. You will have plenty of time to welcome your child, but during the expulsion of the placenta, several minutes later, you will have the choice to be in a position that suits you. You may prefer to stand where gravity once again can assist with the process and the placenta literally falls out. When the cord stops pulsating, your baby will be breathing independently and the cord can then be clamped and cut without any rush or your baby being forced to gasp for its first breath. Even in childbirth it is beneficial to apply the Alexander principle of inhibition rather than have the process rushed, which may lead to the possibility of complications arising.

Feeding

When it comes to feeding your baby, your body knows exactly what to provide; the structure and composition of your own breastmilk has been designed perfectly for a human infant. Breastfeeding activates a series of reflexes in the body: putting your newborn to the breast soon after it is born can actually help to prevent haemorrhaging, as the action of sucking causes the uterus to contract and reduces the flow of blood. It also helps to establish the bond between mother and child, and the antibodies contained in breastmilk help to build up the child's immune system.

It is only in recent times that bottle-feeding has become more popular, partly due to the fact that many women are obliged to return to work within a few weeks of giving birth to their baby. I was amazed recently to hear at a post-natal class that over half the mothers with babies less than six weeks old were already back at full-time work. This was having serious repercussions for both mother and child as their natural instincts were being ignored, and most mothers who were back at work reported that their babies cried frequently and refused to be comforted, which was putting an enormous strain on their relationship with their partner. This illustrates the 'end-gaining' attitude that many of us seem to have adopted today.

Breastfeeding can also save many hours of the new mother's precious time which might otherwise be spent in the preparation, cleaning and sterilization involved in the process of bottle-feeding. Also, because breastmilk is available all the time, your baby does not have to wait – often screaming – to be fed, which can be stressful for both the mother and child.

The most important thing when it comes to feeding is that the mother pauses (inhibits) before making her decision, rather than opting for whatever the current trend may be. Although in some instances breastfeeding will not actually be possible for medical reasons, if the mother is able to choose, she should trust her instincts and choose what she feels is best for herself and her child.

Getting comfortable

It is important that you find a comfortable position in which to feed your baby, as you may be there for half an hour or more at a time. Lying down on your side can be a good position, as it gives you a rest at the same time. If you are sitting up, a bulky cushion behind your back will give you support and help you to sit upright. Make sure that you have another, smaller cushion under the baby's head, as this will bring the baby to you rather than encouraging you to stoop while feeding. If the knee that is under the baby's head is higher than your other knee, this will also give you support – just place your foot on a low stool, a bean-bag or even a pile of books *(see below)*.

Do not forget to apply your directions – it can be helpful to think of lengthening up the front and widening your shoulders, as this will prevent the common habit of hunching or slumping over your baby which gives rise to back, shoulder and neck pain. Make sure you

have a drink nearby, as you may become very thirsty. New mothers are often tense for fear of dropping their baby, and this tension is transmitted to the child and can cause him or her to become agitated. The Alexander Technique can help you to be more aware of this tension when it arises; as soon as you realize that your muscles are tense you can help to let them go by thinking of them relaxing. Unless you are aware of this tension you will not be able to let it go.

The Alexander Technique can also be beneficial to you and your baby by making you

Below. *Mothers can often be seen hunching over their babies when they are feeding them. Since this position is adopted for many hours a week it can lead to tense neck and back muscles which become very uncomfortable. This discomfort can make you irritable and these feelings will be transmitted to your infant.*

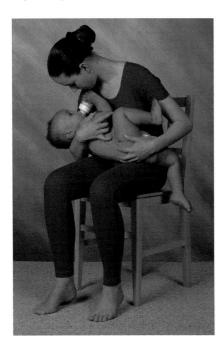

Right. *Whether breastfeeding or bottle-feeding your baby, it is important to take a few moments to get comfortable. Having your foot on a cushion and a pillow under the baby will bring your baby closer to you, which will help to prevent you from developing rounded shoulders and a bent back.*

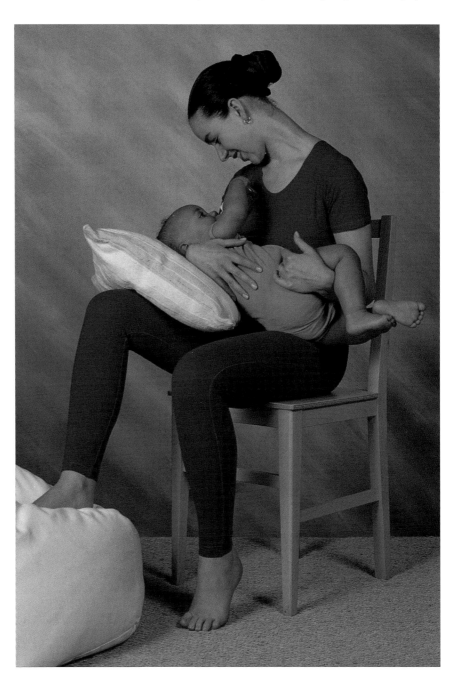

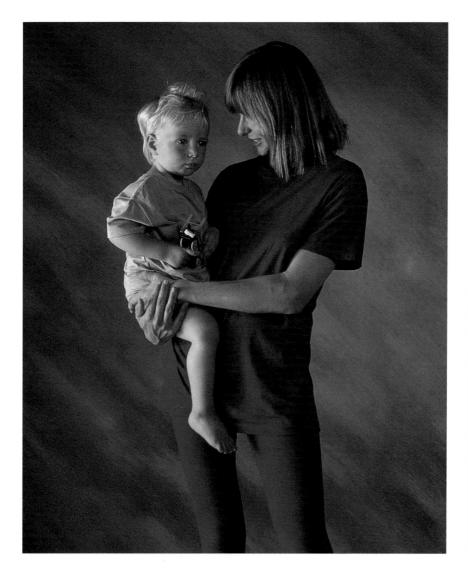

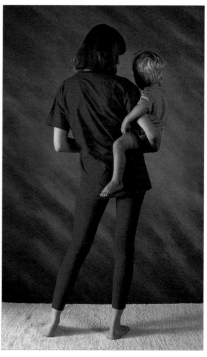

Left and below. *A common way of holding a child is to stand with most of your weight on one leg and use your hip as a 'seat' for the child. This will obviously affect your body alignment as your spine is pulled over to one side. This is a common reason why many parents suffer with backache and neck tension after carrying their children.*

aware of harmful feeding and carrying habits that so easily develop. By thinking of the way you hold your child, you will naturally have more confidence and therefore have less tension which your baby will automatically respond to *(see above and opposite)*.

Be prepared

Pregnancy is one of the most important times in your life, as you are physically and emotionally caring for a new life within your body. It is vital, even in the early stages, for you to be as conscious as possible of the incredible process that is taking place, as this will benefit both you and your unborn child. One of the best ways that you can look after yourself and your baby is to have a course of Alexander lessons, as this will help you to prepare yourself (not only physically, but also mentally and emotionally) for giving life to another human being. Although this can be a very joyful and exciting time, it can also be very draining and demanding on your body, as well as your mind and your emotions. Alexander lessons will stand you in good stead so that you are more able to deal with the stresses and strains that life presents during your pregnancy, childbirth and the early years of motherhood.

The Alexander Technique is a very powerful tool which enables parents to have more choice and less stress in one of the most important experiences of their lives. Releasing tension can help the woman's body to cope with the very powerful changes that take place. It can also help to give your child a less traumatic start in life.

Below. *Here you can clearly see how all this child's weight rests heavily on his mother's left hip. The adjustments that she has to make to her stance in order to compensate for the extra weight will most likely cause aches and pains throughout her body if this position is regularly adopted.*

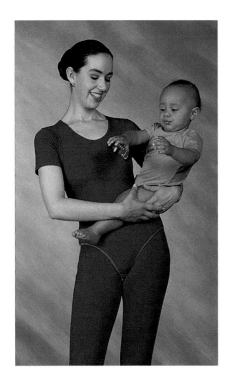

Right. *A better way of holding your baby is to have your weight evenly distributed on both feet and to use your arm as a sling under your child to support its weight. As a result your muscles will be less strained and your baby will feel more secure.*

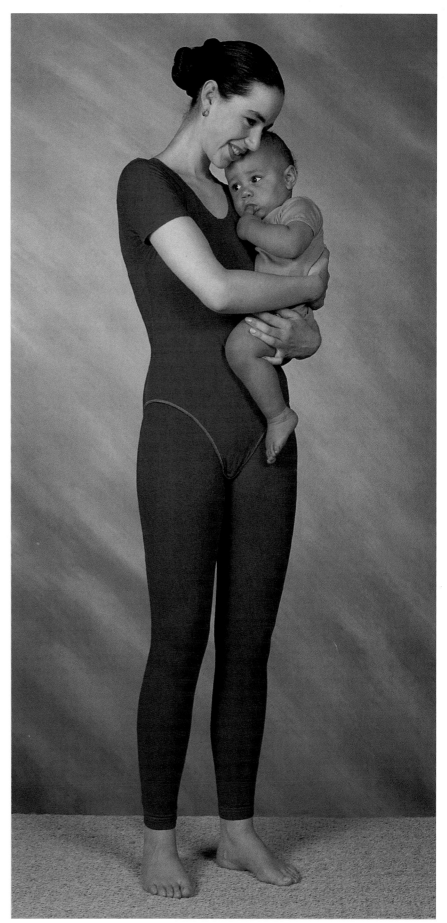

119

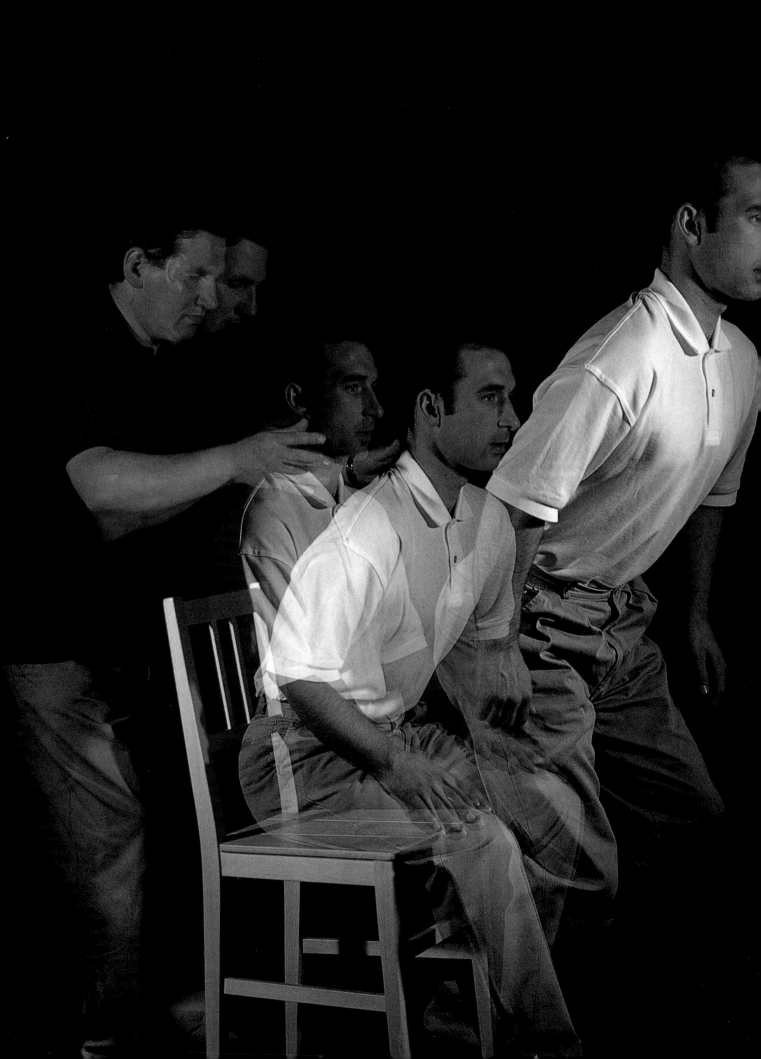

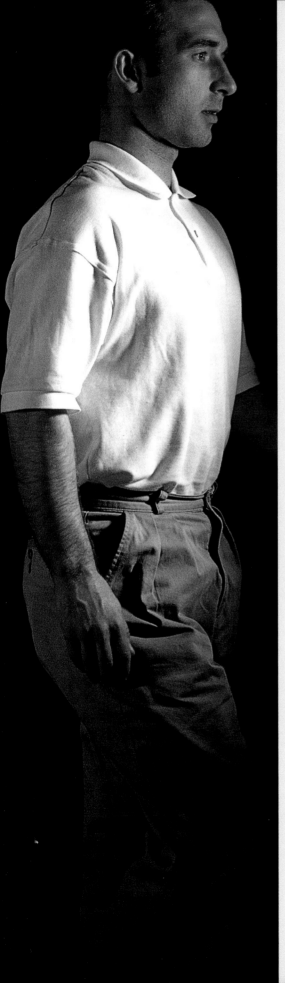

CHAPTER EIGHT

What to expect from an Alexander lesson

*'No man can reveal to you aught,
but that which already lies half asleep in the
dawning of your knowledge.*

*The teacher who walks in the shadow
of the temple, among his followers, gives not
of his wisdom but rather of his faith
and his lovingness.*

*If he is indeed wise he does not bid you enter
the house of his wisdom, but rather leads
you to the threshold of your own mind.'*

Kahil Gibran

*Your Alexander teacher will gently guide your body
through new movements. As the head is directed forward and
up, the spine can lengthen, producing a feeling of lightness – the
hallmark of the Technique. By repeating the same movement
many times you will be able to release the tension by yourself,
giving you greater control over your body.*

What to expect from an Alexander lesson

Although it can be helpful in the first instance to learn the principles and philosophy of the Alexander Technique in groups (such as through attending evening classes or weekend courses), this does not take the place of individual lessons, where a deeper understanding of the Technique can be more easily achieved. Each one of us is unique and therefore we also have unique habits to recognize and let go of.

The length of a lesson varies from teacher to teacher, but on average each will last for between thirty and forty-five minutes. This is because most students can only maintain the level of attention required for the changes to take place for this length of time. The number of lessons needed can vary dramatically from person to person, depending on how ingrained your physical or emotional habits are, as well as on what you are hoping to achieve from the lessons.

A basic course consists of between twenty and thirty lessons. For the first two or three weeks you may find it advantageous to have two lessons a week, but later on when you are more familiar with the principles of the Technique you will be able to apply them on your own, and you may only need a lesson once every two to three weeks. Again, the costs of courses vary, but a whole course rarely costs more than what many people would pay for a holiday, for example. Also, the expense will probably be spread over a year, and can be considerably less than that involved in learning to drive or in a year's maintenance on a car, which many of us can afford. We would not question the validity of keeping our car in good working order by having it serviced, and yet when it comes to our own body we often fail to pay it any attention until the damage has been done.

What takes place during an Alexander lesson will vary depending on your own requirements and the way your teacher chooses to put across the information. If the teacher has not been personally recommended by a friend, it is worth having one lesson from two or three different teachers to see which will suit you best. Various organizations will supply a list of qualified teachers, and their details are listed in the 'useful addresses' section at the back of the book *(see page 141)*.

Since teachers have different styles of teaching, the following account of an Alexander lesson is an approximate guide based on my own experience.

Your first lesson

Your first lesson may be slightly longer than subsequent lessons, and some teachers will ask you to book a double lesson. You may be asked about the state of your health in general and whether you have any medical problems, and your teacher may also want to know why you have come for lessons and what your expectations are. You do not have to have anything wrong with you to benefit from the Technique, but if you do it would be helpful at this point to mention any accident or trauma that you feel might have contributed to any pain or condition from which you may be suffering. Some teachers also take a few minutes to discuss the principles and history behind the Technique.

After this, your teacher may gently move your limbs or head and ask you not to help while he or she checks your body for excessive muscle tension or inappropriate habits. This may be done while you are sitting, standing or lying on a treatment table. At the end of your first session your teacher will advise you as to how many lessons you are likely to need and how often you need to come.

The hardest aspect of an Alexander lesson to communicate in words is the feeling that people have: the experience of the Alexander Technique can never be described in a book or conveyed by speech. It is a wonderful feeling of lightness and ease that allows all parts of the body to work in unison with each other. It gives many people a sense of peace and oneness that they had forgotten was possible. Some people describe the feeling as 'walking on air', or 'having all their joints well oiled'; it is simply the feeling of letting your body work as nature intended without the interference that is practically universal in Western society today. Although the experience can differ for each individual, many people describe it as a weightless sensation, or as though all their worries have been suddenly lifted off their shoulders. One of my students poetically described it as 'the champagne feeling'. Following your first lesson this feeling may only last for a short time after the lesson finishes, but with subsequent lessons this will last for longer and longer periods.

Subsequent lessons

When you have learned how to let go of the existing muscle tension that has accumulated in your body over the years, you will begin to learn various movements that will help to prevent the tension from returning. You will relearn ways of walking, standing, sitting and bending that put less strain on your body. If you are a musician, a sportsperson or have an occupation that is causing specific problems, your teacher can help you to carry out those activities differently, so that you can readjust the movements in order to eliminate pain or improve your performance.

Turn to the following pages to discover some of the ways in which your teacher will show you how the Technique can help you in your daily life.

A 'whole' treatment

It was the philosopher Plato who wisely said that the cure of parts of the body should not be attempted without the treatment of the whole person, which includes the body, emotions, mind and spirit. This was over two thousand years ago, and yet we still try to cure specific parts of the body with our drugs and operations, blindly missing the connections

between physical, mental and emotional well-being. The Alexander Technique not only treats the body as a whole, but it also helps students to change both their mental and emotional outlook on life.

The inner spontaneity that each of us carries around needs to be set free in order for our true potential to shine through, otherwise as soon as we have eradicated one set of symptoms they will appear in a different form elsewhere in the body. We need to find the source of our difficulties and re-programme our conditioned responses so that we are able to live the kind of life we not only deserve, but which is our inherent birthright.

The case histories on pages 134–137 are true accounts from people who have had direct experience of the Technique, written down in their own words.

HOW LESSONS HELP

Although you can read about the principles of the Technique in a book, the best way to understand what is really being asked of you is to have a course of lessons to start off with. The first-hand experience between teacher and student is invaluable in helping you to detect areas of tension within your own body, as well as showing you the harmful habits that you have built up over the years. Lessons help particularly in showing you how to do the following:

• *Release unwanted muscular tension within the body, which helps to relieve or prevent numerous physical ailments including backache, headaches and migraines, neck and shoulder problems and digestive disorders.*
• *Become more conscious of your habitual patterns of behaviour, thus allowing you to make more appropriate decisions.*
• *Prevent premature – and unnecessary – wear and tear on your bones and joints, so helping you to avoid problems normally regarded as age-related, such as osteo-arthritis.*
• *Improve your breathing, which can help with asthma and other respiratory problems.*
• *Conserve your energy by performing actions with the minimum amount of effort.*
• *Rediscover your inherent natural poise and graceful movement that allows you to move through life with greater ease.*

Releasing tension while sitting on a chair

Many of us hold a great deal of tension in our shoulders and arms, and this is often exacerbated if we have a sedentary job in which we spend most of the day hunched over a desk or peering forward to look at a computer screen. Conversely, when we 'sit up straight' we tend to arch our back, causing our body to be tense or sometimes even rigid. This tension is present in every muscle in the body, and can give rise to a whole range of aches and pains.

During Alexander lessons, your teacher will help you to release this tension so that the chair and the floor are supporting you rather than your own tension. It is helpful to remember that when the back lengthens as the head is released forward and upward, the tail bone releases downwards on to the chair, which allows the spine to support the rest of the body naturally. Whenever possible, it is beneficial to have both feet flat on the floor, otherwise your back muscles will have to tense to support the weight of your legs and this will affect your posture. Try not to habitually lean back on to the chair or rely on any supports outside of yourself.

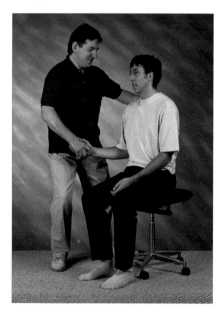

Above and right. *Your teacher will gently move your arms into various positions and when he can feel the tension he will ask you to release it by thinking of lengthening your arm away from your shoulder. You may feel your arm physically growing, which can be a peculiar experience when it first happens, but afterwards your arms will have a wonderful feeling of lightness.*

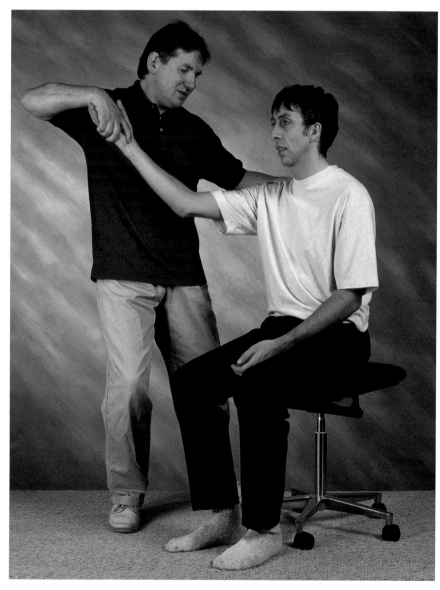

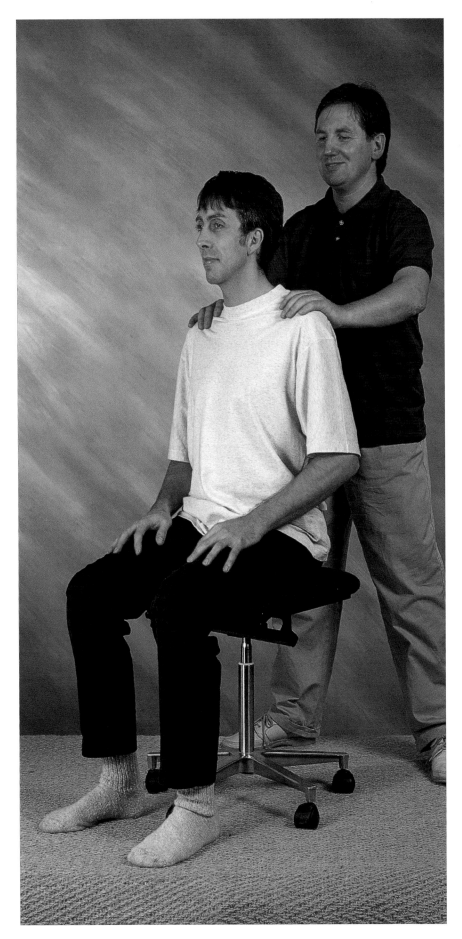

Left. *Here the teacher is helping the student to release the tension that is causing his shoulders to hunch. It is very common for people under stress to draw their shoulders up towards their ears. The teacher's hands are gently laid upon the shoulders and he directs his hands away from one another.*

Below. *The teacher will help you to release the knee from the pelvis, which frees the tension around the hip joint. At the same time he may ask you to think of your shoulder releasing from your knee, which will help the pectoral (chest) muscles to lengthen.*

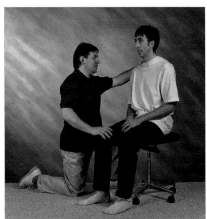

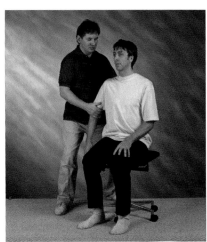

Above. *Here, the teacher's hands help to release any tension in the upper arm as well as under the armpit. This position also has the effect of releasing the chest muscles, which allows the shoulder to extend away from the opposite hip.*

125

Moving from sitting to standing

After a while your teacher will take you into simple everyday movements like getting up from a chair – this is to help you become aware of how you unnecessarily tense your muscles in the process. It is all too easy to react with tension during a simple movement such as this. This stimulates the 'fear reflex', causing you to pull your head back on to your spine, which will, in effect, prevent you from getting up. As a result, you have to push hard with your leg muscles just to move into a standing position.

Your teacher will help you to inhibit this reaction so that you have time to apply your directions – in turn, this will help you to move out of the chair effortlessly. By simply allowing the head to be free from the spine, the head will naturally want to go forward and up. This encourages the spine to elongate, so that even before you start to get up from the chair you are already moving in the right direction. This will help your muscles to remain in a comparative state of rest throughout the movement.

Below. *Your teacher will ask you to inhibit your urge to get up straight away, which gives you a chance to think of your primary directions. Here, the teacher is helping the student to free his neck muscles so that there is freedom between his head and spine.*

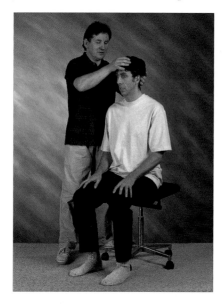

Right. *Using his hands, he will gently guide you into standing and monitor whether or not you are tensing your neck muscles and pulling your head back. If he feels the head retracting, he will ask you again to reinforce the thought of allowing the head to release in a forward and upward direction.*

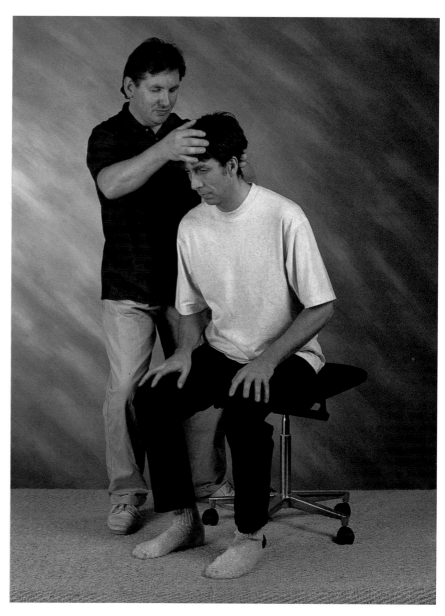

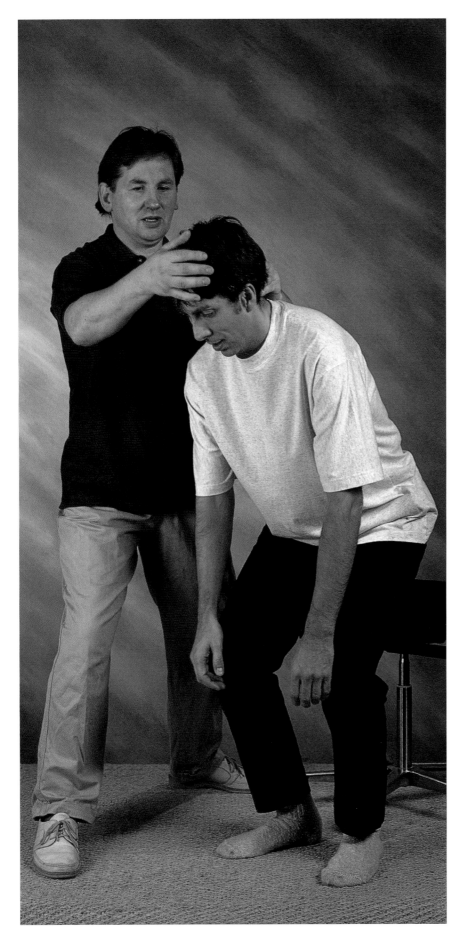

Left. *The teacher's hands will stay with you throughout the entire movement and he will keep encouraging you to lead the movement with your head – he may take you through this movement again and again until you get used to it. At first this new way of getting up may feel strange, but after a while you will get accustomed to it. Notice how the student is encouraged to let his arms hang down freely; this is so he is not pushing down on his legs and creating excess tension counter to the direction in which he is moving.*

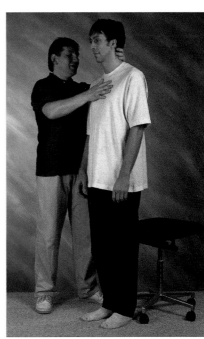

Above. *When you finally reach the standing position, your teacher will continue to help you to release muscular tension by still encouraging you to think of freedom in the neck. This allows your head to go forward and up, so elongating the spine. Here, the teacher is also helping the student to release up in the front of his body rather than pull down, which is what many people tend to do.*

127

Moving from standing into walking

Many people walk with far more tension than they really need, partly because they are often in a hurry to get somewhere and partly because they are not walking in the way that nature intended. Many of us think that walking consists of picking up one leg, with all the tension that that entails – each leg weighs approximately 8.5 kg (1½ stone) – and then displacing our weight on to our other leg, so placing the hip joint under considerable strain. We then place our other leg in front of our body once more and repeat this process – this, we think, is walking.

To walk with grace and ease, so that none of our muscles or joints are placed under undue stress, we need to look towards the direction in which we wish to go, and as we release our neck muscles the head will naturally go forward, which results in a 'falling forward' movement. As we do this, more weight is thrown on to the toes, which triggers off the reflexes in the feet, and each step is then taken automatically. It is important to realize that the action of walking is controlled by the reflexes, and therefore can be done without any effort on our part.

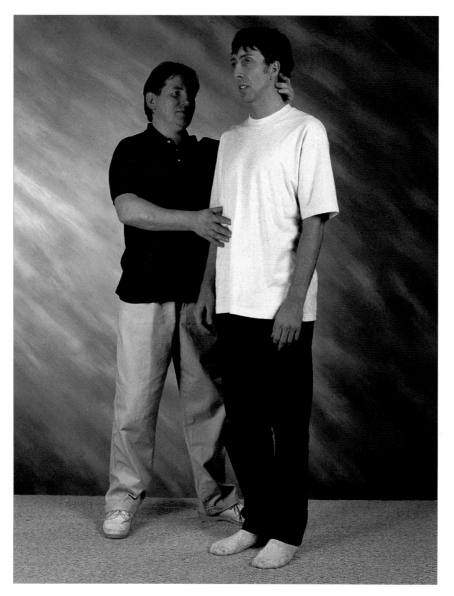

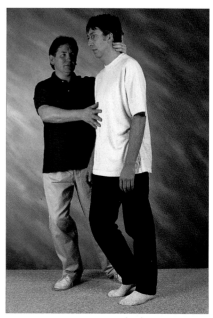

Left. *Your Alexander teacher will use his hands again to help you to lengthen from your feet up to the top of your head. You may even feel yourself growing, which is exactly what is happening! Initially, this may make you feel very unstable compared to your usual posture.*

Above. *This man's body is now more unstable and therefore is able to move more easily. Just thinking of freeing the neck allows his head to go slightly forward, which causes his entire body to go out of balance, and he begins to move forward effortlessly.*

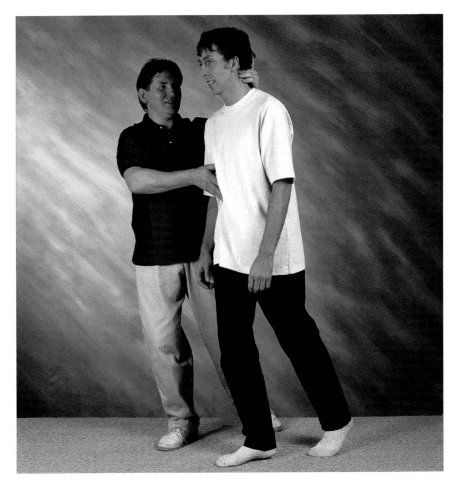

Left. This student's sensory reflex system perceives that his body is falling forward and his leg and foot automatically step forward to regain his balance. This sequence of events is repeated several times and results in the action of walking. Throughout the movement, the teacher's hands encourage the student's neck to be free and the muscles in the front of the body to lengthen.

Below. Here the teacher is encouraging more flexibility in the hip, knee and ankle joints by taking the student into a squat. The teacher helps to keep the back aligned so that the entire body is in balance. If there is equal weight both behind and in front of the feet, the muscles do not have to tense in order to support the body.

Picking up an object

Your teacher will also guide you through everyday actions to help you relearn movements that your body has forgotten how to perform correctly. Picking up an object is something that we all do many times a day, yet we often bend from the waist, keeping our legs braced back with our knee and ankle joints completely tense. This places the back muscles under an enormous strain because they are supporting most of the weight of the body in order to prevent it from falling forwards.

It is far kinder to the body to bend at the hip, knee and ankle joints, as these are designed specifically for this purpose – to take the body up and down. Children use these joints naturally without thought, and they often adopt a squatting position which they can comfortably maintain for long periods of time. But as children we tend to copy our parents, and gradually squatting begins to feel alien to us; yet it is far kinder on our body.

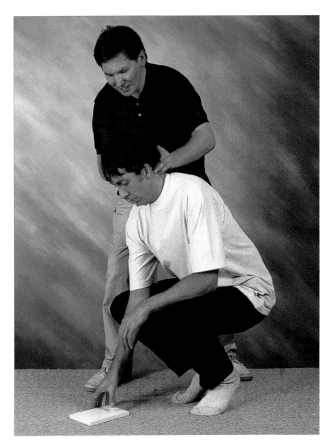

Releasing tension while lying down

It is easier to release tension while lying down because the body's muscular system is not involved in having to keep you upright. Also, you do not have the same fear of falling over when lying down. Some teachers like to use the table a great deal, while others only use it during the first few lessons. A table session can have the effect of the muscles releasing in a short space of time, so you may find that when you get off the table you are slightly disorientated for a few moments while your body adjusts to its new height and sense of freedom. You will gradually become accustomed to this feeling as your lessons progress, and it will soon feel completely natural – in fact, you will probably forget how much tension you used to carry within your body all the time. While you are lying down you will have the added advantage of the spine lengthening more quickly than when standing or sitting, which will assist in releasing the tension throughout the rest of your body.

Right. *Here the Alexander teacher gently takes the student's leg up towards his chest to increase the flexibility of the pelvic joint. This also has the effect of lengthening the muscle in his lower back and releasing the tension that is so often responsible for back pain.*

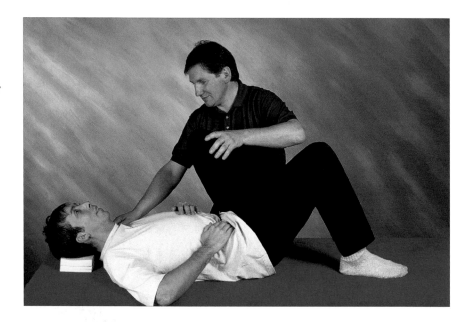

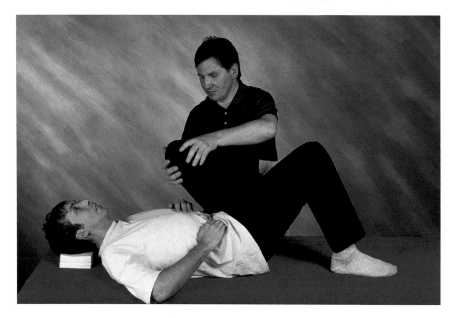

Left. *As the teacher takes the student's leg further up towards his chest he is careful not to use any force, and much of the movement comes from the student's own ability to release tension. This movement encourages the back muscles to lengthen further still, without placing them under any excessive strain.*

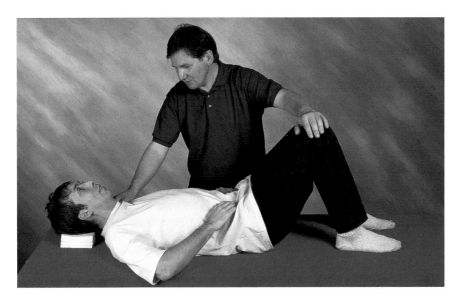

Left. *Here the teacher is helping his student to allow his shoulder to lengthen away from the opposite hip while he thinks of his directions. This will release the muscles that often spiral around the torso.*

Below. *The teacher needs to think of his own directions, both primary and secondary, and the feeling of calmness and relaxation is transmitted to the student by both touch and the teacher's presence of stillness. Here the student is allowing his arm to extend, which releases tension in his shoulder and back.*

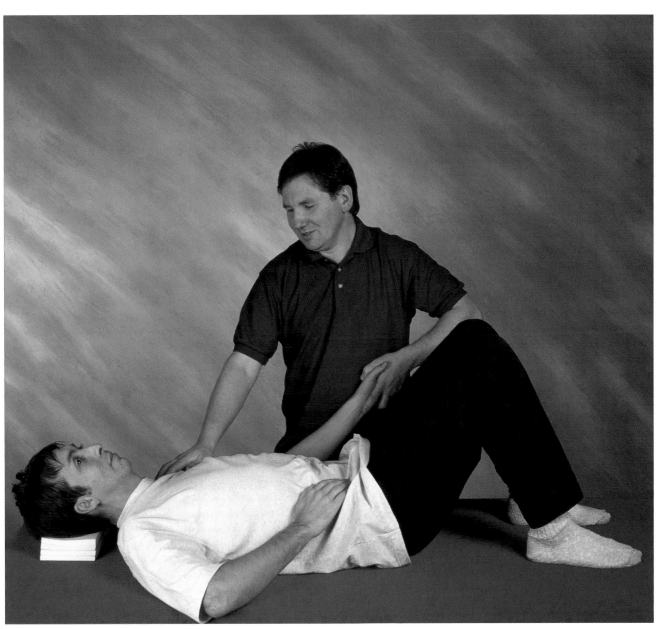

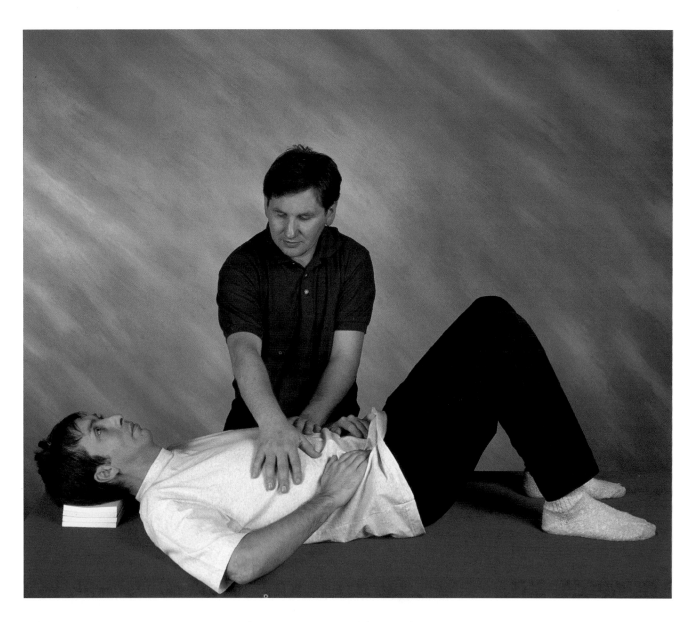

Above. *The teacher helps his student to release the muscles surrounding the rib-cage. This will encourage deeper and more efficient breathing. It is amazing how many people use only a fraction of their lung capacity when they breathe; as a result they are prone to tire easily. They also tend to feel less enthusiastic about life in general, and are likely to take longer to recover from illnesses.*

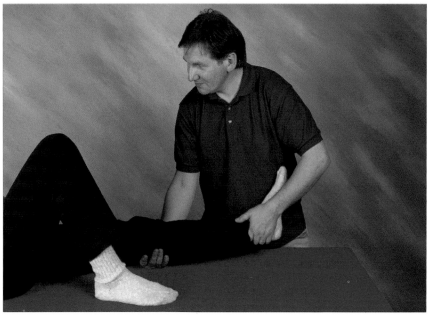

Left. *Here the teacher is helping his student to release the tension in the leg and pelvic muscles. The teacher directs the student's leg away from his torso, and it is not unusual to see the leg actually elongate by 2–3 cm (1 in) or even more.*

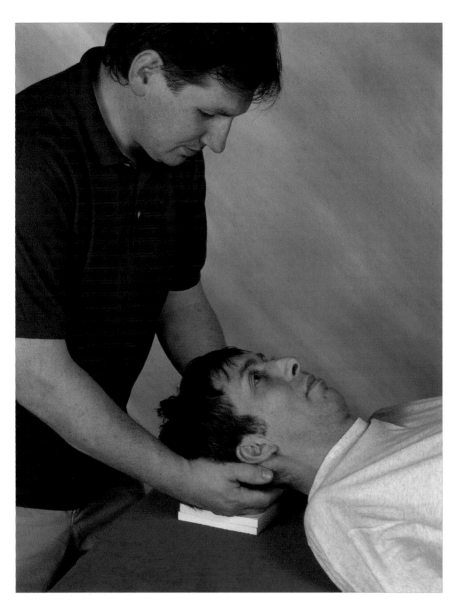

Left. *When lying down it is easier to let go of tension in the neck muscles by allowing the teacher to support your head. This encourages more freedom between the skull and the top vertebra (the atlas), which in turn allows the rest of the spine to lengthen.*

Below far left. *Here the teacher is directing the student's shoulders away from one another. This helps to release tension in the upper chest, which encourages deeper breathing and also allows the shoulders to release backward so that the shoulder blades are more in contact with the ribs. This will encourage the student to have more confidence and will promote a greater sense of well-being.*

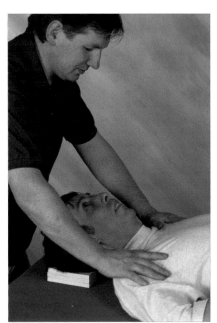
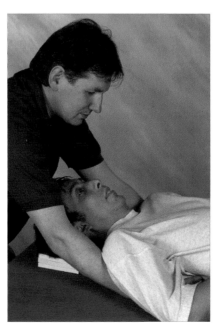

Left. *Here the teacher has his hands under the shoulder blades and he is directing his hands towards the head. This will have the effect of lengthening the student's back – the lumbar region flattens out and makes more contact with the table naturally. The spine can then be more supportive, rather than the body's activity muscles having to do all the work. The student may also find that he is a little taller when he gets off the table.*

Case histories

Name: Kim Wells
Occupation: Lawyer
Age: 33

I had heard from a friend that the Alexander Technique had helped her painful back as well as improving her posture. Since both my parents were back sufferers and I tended also to suffer from back pain from time to time, I thought it would be a good idea to try the Alexander Technique in the hope that it would prevent the problem from getting any worse. I also wanted to improve my posture, because years of bending over desks studying and, more recently, working had caused me to feel that I had become a little round-shouldered. It was not unusual for me to leave the office with agonizing neckache, and I was aware that, if faced with a situation in which I felt particularly self-conscious, my shoulders would become even more rounded.

When I arrived for my first lesson I did not know what to expect at all. After a brief introduction, my teacher helped me to relax and to become more aware of my movements, and I was very surprised to find that by the end of my lesson I felt very different. I had a lovely feeling of lightness and ease throughout my whole body; I went home and described it to my husband as feeling as though I was walking on the moon. I was afraid that if I sat down I would lose the wonderful feeling and I wanted to enjoy this new-found freedom for as long as possible. I could not remember ever feeling so free of tension.

As the lessons progressed I began to notice that it was not just my body that felt different. I was less stressed at work and I gradually became much more confident and able to deal with other sides of my life more competently. Although I did not feel such a dramatic difference in the subsequent lessons, the tension in my neck gradually eased and I started to have a far more positive outlook on life, which helped me to enjoy my work more.

I would not say that these days I never suffer from tension because I am in a fairly stressful occupation and there are many different demands made on me during a working day. However, I am much more aware of when the tension is beginning and I have learned to do something about it myself. The Alexander Technique helps me to cope with the problems that arise every day, without feeling overwhelmed at any time. I am able to organize my day much more efficiently and I am able to look ahead and stop to reflect. Just stopping for a moment before I answer the telephone, for instance, enables me to clarify my thoughts. I meet a lot of people through my work and I am sure that because I feel more relaxed I am able to project myself better, which increases my confidence.

This new confidence has also affected my life outside the office – I have recently taken up amateur dramatics and, although going on stage is extremely nerve-racking, by being able to relax and feel assured I am able to enjoy performing. I have become more outgoing since discovering the Technique and I play more sport than I used to, in particular rediscovering tennis and taking up horse riding for the first time. I can honestly say that I am now getting much more enjoyment out of life.

Since seeing the changes in me, my husband, also a lawyer, has taken up the Alexander Technique and has also benefited greatly from it. Many people in my profession do tend to suffer from tension, backaches and various stress-related problems, and I have absolutely no hesitation in recommending the Alexander Technique to them.

Name: Paul Stone
Occupation: Doctor
Age: 32

As a doctor I became aware of the effect one's mind has on one's health and well-being, and through my work I realized that it was 'disease' of the mind that directly caused many of the illnesses I was treating, rather than actual physical symptoms. Part of my work consisted of health education in the community (working with children and their families), as well as a degree of involvement with mental health projects, so I was coming into contact with patients across the board.

It was seeing so much illness and suffering that made me determined that I was not going to let my body get old before its time – so I took up running. When I first started to run I felt a new power, freedom and confidence. This freedom was complemented by being amongst nature in the open air, running on grass, surrounded by plants, birds and blue sky, in the sun, wind and snow. Running soon became a passion I shared with other club members. We ran for fun as well as in charity events around the world. It was not long, however, before I began to get pain in my knee joints and my body began to get increasingly uncomfortable. I had heard of the Alexander Technique and was now drawn to it because it covered not only physical but also psychological development. I started to have lessons straight away.

This new knowledge of how the body works in movement helped me in my warm-ups as well as while I was actually running. I soon realized that while running I was pulling my head back because my neck muscles were over-tightened, and my chest was thrusting forward, causing my shoulder blades to be pushed towards each other. I also noticed that my shoulders were hunched, causing a great deal of tension in my arms which led to very rigid wrists and elbows. As I learned more about myself through the Technique, I also detected that I was only breathing in the top part of my lungs, my fists were often clenched unnecessarily and I was even pushing my hips forward.

After some time I started to put the principles of the Alexander Technique into practice, which greatly improved my running. The lessons to that point had helped me to improve my balance and co-ordination and I soon learned how to release much of the tension as I ran. By thinking of my new directions I was able to stop pulling my head back on to my spine, and this alone brought my whole body back into balance; I was able to lead with my head and this consequently allowed my spine to lengthen. I could feel my rib-cage release, and my breathing became deeper and more controlled. I also thought of my back widening, which prevented my shoulder blades from being pushed together, and as a result my shoulders and arms became more relaxed so they naturally started to swing more freely. The pain in my knee gradually faded with time.

At first, my new way of running felt odd, even awkward, but I soon became used to the changes and reorganization to which my entire muscular system was being subjected. Through perseverance my body adopted a new sensation of lightness as every joint seemed to have more freedom. Greater speed, longer distances, fewer injuries and a much smoother style were my reward.

It is not uncommon for many runners to trip and fall when running over uneven surfaces. As a result of my increased awareness, suppleness and ability to react more quickly, I now fall on fewer occasions, and when I do I fall more gracefully, decreasing the chances of serious injury. I now find that I am able to run with greater ease and far less effort than before, and can run further with less wasted energy. I also enjoy my running much more than ever before. The Alexander Technique has proved to be an invaluable tool in this respect, as well as helping in many other areas of my life.

From an emotional point of view, I used to be easily knocked off balance by unexpected events in my life and, although I put on a brave face, I lacked confidence and often became upset over little things. The process I went through while learning the Technique was one of consciously reclaiming myself – physically, emotionally and mentally. I now feel much calmer, more flexible and much more sure of what I want in life. It has enhanced my natural spontaneity and enthusiasm for living. I am much more aware of when I am under pressure and I am able to check the build-up of tension when it occurs. This allows me to be in control when difficult situations arise, and to deal with any problems in a constructive way. The Alexander Technique is also of great benefit in my work as a doctor, because I am able to prevent the pressures of my job interfering with my relationship with my patients.

Name: Jo Howard
Occupation: Horse Breeder and Trainer
Riding Instructor
Age: 49

I had heard of the Alexander Technique frequently during the course of my work from several different sources, but had found it very difficult to know who to approach. I had immediately been attracted to the Technique and I knew it was something I wanted to find out more about, even though I had no idea what it entailed. Eventually I discovered some books on the subject and decided to go on a five-day introductory course.

At the time I was at a very low point in my life, and was suffering with acute depression, chronic back pain and colon problems. I was also in agony with neckache, which felt like a steel rod going up into my neck producing frequent headaches and migraines. I cannot adequately describe the sheer misery I was experiencing.

I had been analyzing myself for two years trying to understand why I was so successful in business and such a failure in my personal life. I was questioning all the things I had acquired in life and wondering why these material possessions were not making me happy. I knew deep down that things were not right, but I did not know why. I had a very strong sense that there was more to life than what I was experiencing, and in actual fact there was more to *me* than I was aware of. I had become very low and had got no self-esteem – and I mean *no* self-esteem whatsoever; I did not know how to begin to get

back my self-confidence. It took all my will power and courage even to pick up the phone and make that first call to an Alexander teacher to ask for help, and even more courage to travel the hundred miles to where the course was being held.

I found that the benefits from that initial five-day course were enormous – it changed my whole perception of myself. I could not believe how much my life had altered in such a short time, and that something so gentle could actually be so powerful. I returned home with tools that I could use in order to transform my life and with a determination that I wanted to take it further in the form of private lessons, which I did.

As the lessons progressed I became increasingly aware that I was holding on to a whole lifetime of tension without realizing it; I started moving differently, which also greatly improved my balance and co-ordination while riding horses. All my aches and pains gradually disappeared and I began to be able to change my mental attitudes to life. Over the course of the past two-and-a-half years (since starting Alexander lessons) I have not had one headache or migraine, which I am amazed by. My back hurts momentarily if I twist or turn awkwardly, but the constant tormenting pain that I experienced for years has gone completely.

The process has felt like stripping away layer upon layer of outworn conditioning, which I was unaware that I was carrying, in the form of old attitudes and unexpressed emotions. I have discovered the real me underneath it all and this is what I had been denying. The whole experience has been a major life-change for me: I feel that I have made leaps in my personal growth; I feel totally different about myself; and I now have self-esteem whereas I used to have none. I have found the confidence to do things that three years ago I would not have thought possible. Most of all, it has helped me to claim the right just to be myself without the feelings of worry or guilt that I so often carried around. Also, with my new-found confidence I have grown in height by two inches!

Name: Mary Wright
Occupation: Retired Secretary
Age: 77

My problems started when I was fourteen years old. I remember it clearly: I was sitting on the floor at school one afternoon when another child accidentally trod on my left leg – the pain was excruciating. I walked with a limp for a few weeks afterwards, but received no treatment for the injury. After a time the pain began to abate, but I now realize that I had got into the habit of walking with more weight on my right leg.

Since my early thirties I have always suffered with neck and back pain and was only offered pain-killing drugs as a solution; these pains were apparently normal for anyone in my line of work. My doctor informed me that it was arthritis, which was due to excessive wear and tear of my bones; he told me that there was nothing I could do and that I would just have to learn to live with it.

Over the last forty years the pain increased and it affected everything that I did. It made me bad-tempered, and I often used to lose my temper with other members of my family and feel very guilty afterwards. I also suffered from high blood pressure and insomnia; it was not unusual for me to wake up four or five times a night.

One day my son, who is a musician, mentioned the Alexander Technique to me, and said that he was going to start having lessons because of a recurring pain in his shoulder. After some weeks I began to notice a change in him – he seemed to be altering his shape! It was most uncanny, but with his new posture came a sense of contentment and greater confidence. I was so intrigued that I decided to have a lesson myself.

After my first lesson I came away with a strange sensation in my left leg – it was as if my teacher had twisted my leg by ninety degrees, but I could see for myself that it was perfectly straight! He pointed out that I had formed a habit of turning my left foot inwards and this was throwing my body out of balance, causing tension in my back and neck. During the subsequent lessons this new way of moving began to feel less strange and I could feel that I was walking in a more upright manner. I could also feel that I was growing and regaining the height that I had lost in recent years.

It has now been a year since my first lesson and I cannot believe the change in my life in that time. I am moving with fluidity and an ease that I had not thought possible; I am now striding through the shopping centre rather than walking with my old shuffle! I no longer have any trouble sleeping at night, the pains in my back and neck have gradually disappeared and my blood pressure has dropped. The most noticeable change, however, is the fact that my whole personality is different. I no longer feel sorry for myself and consequently I am a much happier and less worried person.

I feel very lucky that I am able to enjoy an active retirement when so many of my friends seem to be struggling with so many problems. I have recently taken up travelling again, which is something I never thought I would do at my age. I am deeply indebted to the Alexander Technique for giving me this new lease of life.

Afterword

The Alexander Technique is often thought of as merely a physical technique to improve posture or help eliminate muscle tension that is causing pain or discomfort. As we have seen, the Technique does both of these things; but there are also many other benefits that it brings, of which many people are unaware. Since the body, mind, emotions and spirit are all interconnected and inseparable, when you release physical tensions throughout your body, your mind and emotions are influenced at the same time.

As you become able to use your body more efficiently, you will have more energy to do the things that you enjoy. Often, the tiredness that many of us feel throughout the day or in the evenings is replaced with more energy and enthusiasm, which enables us to achieve more during our day. This naturally gives us a greater sense of fulfilment in our lives, and when the body is more active it is more likely to function naturally, which will maintain it in a better condition in later life.

Mental benefits

Many mental conditions can also be helped by the Technique. If we look at depression, for example, although it is a mental illness we can often recognize a depressed person by the slumped position of their body; in fact, the word 'depressed' is also describing their body shape. If you are able to improve the poise of a person suffering from depression, then it follows that their state of mind may also improve. The same principle applies to worried, insecure or anxious people; by applying the Alexander Technique many people can calm their mind and become more confident, enabling them to face the challenges and changes that life inevitably brings. Worry and anxiety are merely mental habits that have been acquired over the years, and by applying the principles of inhibition and free choice we can also let go of these tendencies.

One of the first things that many people experience after starting Alexander lessons is an improved sleep pattern, and they wake up in the morning feeling more refreshed. Sleep is the body's natural healing and rejuvenating process and it is vital for a balanced, healthy lifestyle. A person's whole attitude to life can change, as they begin to look forward to their day rather than wish their life away. People also report that, although the situation at work or at home may be the same, they no longer feel as stressed and find that they have fewer arguments or conflicts. After a number of lessons it not unusual for some people to experience clearer thoughts, which leads to an improved memory and greater efficiency in general.

It was W. Somerset Maugham who astutely commented, 'It's a funny thing about life; if you refuse to accept anything but the best, you very often get it.' In short, by practising the Technique we are given the ability to enhance our quality of life. If we can consciously choose to say no to the things in our life that cause us stress, we not only improve our own life, but also favourably affect the lives of those around us.

Emotional benefits

In these hectic times when everything has to be done yesterday, our feelings can become so buried that we lose touch with the very important emotional part of our lives. We are living in a dehumanized society where money and social status come before human feelings, and in the pressure of the business world we can often lose touch with our emotional needs. Our dreams and life-goals become lost in our endeavour to achieve them.

Through learning and applying the Alexander Technique you will be able to return to a balanced life where emotions and human values once again have the importance they deserve. This 're-balancing' will enable you to

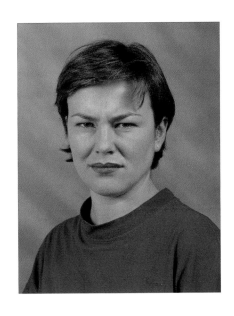

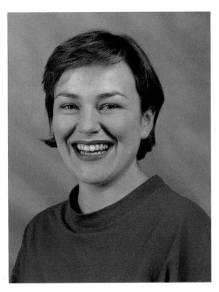

Far left. *When people are under stress or worried, their facial muscles often become very tense and their features become hard, reflecting a cynical or sceptical outlook on life. If this is allowed to continue over many years, muscle tension can begin to distort their face.*

Left. *After Alexander lessons, people naturally feel more contented with their life – their whole face becomes more attractive and their eyes light up and have a clearer, child-like quality. People can often look years younger as the tension in their face melts away.*

replace frustration, anxiety and worry with happiness, peace and contentment. Concern about the future will gradually be replaced by an enjoyment of each day as it comes, and you will begin to appreciate all the precious gifts that you already possess, rather than hankering for material goods or status that you have not yet managed to acquire.

We need to absorb and enjoy each moment as it comes. Our mind can be thinking of the experiences of the past or planning the near or distant future, and our emotions can be experiencing the nostalgia of what has gone or longing for what might be, but our body can never leave the here and now. When we focus on our body through inhibition and direction we will be able to be truly present, and this allows us simply to enjoy *being* in the present moment.

As excessive muscular tension disappears, we often feel that a weight has been lifted off our shoulders and that we can cope better in general; gradually we gain more control of our life. We feel able to express our feelings in a more constructive way, instead of allowing emotions to build up, only to erupt inappropriately at a later date. Past emotions can become trapped within the muscles and, as these release, the emotions are also liberated and we are able to become more balanced. Alexander once said that people translate everything, whether physical, mental or even spiritual, into muscular tension *(see above)*.

In intense discussions or debates, when emotions are running high, the Alexander Technique can be particularly useful. If you can pause for a moment before speaking, you are less likely to say something that you will regret later; you will also have enough time to collect your thoughts and put together sentences that will have more impact and get your message across clearly and concisely. You will also be in a better position to listen to the other person's point of view before judging the situation.

Spiritual benefits

The Alexander Technique heightens your awareness of all things, and a greater sense of peace can be felt in whatever you are doing. The frantic behaviour to which we have become accustomed is left behind and a greater appreciation of life emerges. You will begin to notice sights, sounds and smells to which you have previously been oblivious.

Just consider for a moment what is happening in this very instant. Your eyes are reading these words, but you are also breathing; something is causing your lungs to inhale and exhale, giving you life, and yet this is simply taken for granted. Your breath is quietly giving you life each and every moment, but how often do you really appreciate that quiet miracle that started the instant you were born and continues for every second that you are alive? Behind your every breath is your spirit waiting calmly and patiently to be noticed.

The Alexander Technique not only helps you to be more attentive to yourself, but also to your environment. A greater mindfulness develops as you become more alive and conscious of things of which you were previously unaware. When rushing from place to place, so preoccupied with thoughts, everything around us becomes just a blur. In the artificial environments we have created we often cut ourselves off from nature so effectively that we hardly know what season it is. The awareness that the Alexander Technique brings helps us to slow down to a pace where we can appreciate the beauty of the natural world, and realize that we are part of that world ourselves.

Free choice

By freeing yourself from physical, mental and emotional habits you may begin to be aware of other tendencies which hold you back in life. As children, some of the conditioning that we experience causes us to think and react in ways that are inappropriate, and by recognizing this conditioning we can break our old habits and start to think for ourselves, instead of going along with everyone else.

Many people live their life according to 'should', 'ought to', 'must', 'can't' and 'have to', rather than how they want to. In my opinion, the major cause of stress today is the fact that many people's lives are full of things that they do not want to do, instead of activities that they enjoy doing. The next time you feel stressed, ask yourself, 'Am I doing what I want to do, or am I doing something that I feel I have to do?' If you can increase the number of activities that you want to do, and decrease the number of things about which you feel you have no choice, you will automatically feel less stressed and consequently experience much less muscle tension.

If a person commits a crime we take away their freedom as punishment, yet most people are actually giving up this liberty every day without realizing it. It is only by true conscious choice that we can free ourselves in order to achieve our true potential. Alexander saw his Technique primarily as a way in which to regain the freedom of choice that is our birthright, and which is also the major difference that sets us apart from the rest of the animal kingdom. He was convinced that he had discovered an essential tool that allows us to progress on the evolutionary path towards becoming a greater race of people.

The Alexander Technique, as we have seen, is not merely a postural technique to help you to sit, stand and move with poise and grace – it is, in fact, possibly one of the greatest discoveries of the twentieth century, whose great importance is only beginning to emerge. It is a different way of living that allows every one of us to raise our awareness so that we can understand ourselves more fully and be able to claim our supreme inheritance: our ability to choose *how* we live our lives and make conscious choices that will enable us not only to move through life with greater ease, but also to live life to the full and, above all, enjoy living in the present.

Resources

Useful addresses

Richard Brennan runs three-year teacher training courses throughout England, as well as shorter weekend and week courses. For details on any of these courses please send a stamped addressed envelope to:

The Alexander Technique Training Centre
c/o Richard Brennan
48 St Edward's Road
Southsea, Hants PO5 3DJ
England

For a list of teachers in your area please contact one of the following addresses:

UK
The Society of Teachers of the Alexander Technique
20 London House
266 Fulham Road
London SW10 9EL

Alexander Technique Network
PO Box 53
Kendal
Cumbria LA9 4UP

USA
Alexander Technique International, Inc.
1692 Massachusetts Avenue
Cambridge, MA 02138

The North American Society of Teachers of the Alexander Technique
PO Box 112484
Tacoma
WA 98411–2484

Alexander Technique Workshops (USA)
PO Box 408
Ojai, CA 93024

Canada
The Canadian Society of Teachers of the Alexander Technique
PO Box 47025
Apt. 12
555 West 12th Avenue
Vancouver, BC V5Z 3X0

Australia
The Australian Society of Teachers of the Alexander Technique
PO Box 716
Darlinghurst
NSW 2010

Direction Magazine
(A journal on the Alexander Technique with worldwide subscriptions)
PO Box 276
Bondi
NSW 2026

South Africa
The South African Society of Teachers of the Alexander Technique
35 Thornhill Road
Rondebosch 7700

Further reading

Easy-to-follow and informative books on the Technique:
Brennan, Richard. *The Alexander Technique: Natural Poise for Health.* Shaftesbury, England: Element Books, 1991.
Brennan, Richard. *The Alexander Technique Workbook.* Shaftesbury, England: Element Books, 1992.
Gelb, Michael. *Body Learning.* London: Aurum Press, 1981.

Books by F.M. Alexander himself, which in some parts are technical in content:
Alexander, F. M. *Conscious Control of the Individual.* London: Gollancz, 1987.
Alexander, F. M. *Man's Supreme Inheritance.* Long Beach, CA: Centerline Press, 1988.
Alexander, F. M. *The Universal Constant in Living.* Long Beach, CA: Centerline Press, 1986.
Alexander, F. M. *The Use of the Self.* London: Gollancz, 1985.

Books about living in the present:
Bach, Richard. *Illusions.* London: Pan Books, 1977.
Carnegie, Dale. *How to Stop Worrying and Start Living.* Tadworth, England: Cedar Books, 1962.
Ende, Michael. *Momo.* London/New York: Penguin Books, 1984.
Liedloff, Jean. *The Continuum Concept.* London: Penguin Books, 1975.
Sacks, Oliver. *A Leg to Stand on.* London: Pan Books, 1986.
Wilson, Colin. *Frankenstein's Castle.* Bath, England: Ashgrove Press, 1968.

Interesting books on sport which are related to the Alexander Technique:
Galleway, W. Timothy. *The Inner Game of Tennis.* London: Jonathan Cape Ltd, 1975.
Herrigel, Eugen. *Zen and the Art of Archery.* London: Arkana, 1953.

Books on natural pregnancy and childbirth:
Balaskas, Janet and Gordon, Yehudi. *The Encyclopedia of Pregnancy and Birth.* London/Sydney: Macdonald, 1987.
Balaskas, Janet and Gordon, Yehudi. *Water Birth.* London: Unwin, 1990.
Charlish, Anne. *Your Natural Baby.* Frenchs Forest, Australia: National, 1996.
Charlish, Anne. *Your Natural Pregnancy.* London: Boxtree, 1995.
La Leche League. *The Art of Breastfeeding.* London: Angus & Robertson, 1988.
Verny, Dr Thomas and Kelly, John. *The Secret Life of the Unborn Child.* London: Sphere Books, 1992.

The Alexander self-help tape

This audio cassette is the perfect accompaniment to *The Alexander Technique Manual* and gives clear and concise instructions on:

- *How to eliminate unwanted tension.*
- *How to prevent or relieve back pain.*
- *How to improve your breathing.*
- *How to clear your mind from unwanted thoughts.*
- *How to practise the two Alexander principles of inhibition and direction.*
- *How to stay in the present moment.*

For details, please contact: STAT Books, 20 London House, 266 Fulham Road, London SW10 9EL, England. Please include a stamped addressed envelope.

Wedge cushions

Information about wedge-shaped cushions for improving posture while sitting can be obtained from The Alexander Technique Training Centre *(see useful addresses).* Please include a stamped addressed envelope.

Index

Acknowledgements

I wish to thank the following people for their help in the creation of this book. First to Susan Mears who put forward the idea of me writing once again; to Ian Jackson, Elaine Partington, Zoë Hughes, Tessa Monina and other members of Eddison Sadd whose high standards of excellence have made writing this book a pleasure; to Steve Marwood for his hard work and endless patience during those long photographic sessions; to Barnfield Riding Stables for their kind assistance and loan of facilities; to Sarah Widdicome for proofreading the first draft; to the following models: Sophie Bevan, Ciaran Brennan, Lorraine Geard, Simon Gillies, Mark Gough, Caroline Green, Mia and Iona Hutchinson, Chloë Inman, Ian Jackson, Camilla Mars, Clara Miriam, Nicky Moran, Marc Salnicki, Joshua Somersall-Weekes, Kate Widdicombe and Donna Williams; to Refia Sacks and Nickie Evans R.G.N., R.N., D.P.S.M., for their informative help about childbirth; to Dr Miriam Wohl M.B., CH.B, J.C.C.Cert, for her invaluable advice and friendship while writing this book; and lastly to Caroline my wife for her encouragement and computer support throughout the project.

EDDISON · SADD EDITIONS

Project Editor Zoë Hughes
Editor Tessa Monina
Proofreader Nikky Twyman
Indexer Dorothy Frame

Art Director Elaine Partington
Mac Designer Brazzle Atkins
Assistant Designer Lynne Ross
Illustrator Aziz Khan

Production Hazel Kirkman and Charles James

The photographs on page 11, page 23 and page 46 are reproduced by kind permission of Neil Cooper/Panos Pictures, Direction Journal and Animals Unlimited respectively.